Testicular Cancer, Varicocele, and Testicular Torsion.

Causes, symptoms, and treatment of testicular pain, varicocele, tumor, torsion, spermatocele, hernia, and more. A Patient's Guide.

Dr. Rupert B. Hansen

Dedicated to my dear wife who first encouraged me to (finally) write this book on the topic of testicular diseases and secondly, supported me lovingly throughout the long hours of research and writing that were necessary to put this plan to practice.

Disclaimer and Legal Notice

The author and publisher did their best to collect and present accurate and helpful information and general advice on the different subjects of this book. Nevertheless, the content of this book is only for informational and educational purposes. This book is not meant to be used, nor should it be used, to diagnose or treat any medical condition. For diagnosis or treatment of any medical problem, consult qualified physicians. The publisher and author are not responsible for any specific health or allergy needs that may require medical supervision and are not liable for any damages or negative consequences from any treatment, action, application or preparation, to any person reading or following the information in this book. References are provided for informational purposes only and do not constitute endorsement of any websites or other sources. Readers should be aware that the websites listed in this book may change.

Copyright and Trademarks

Table of Contents

Introduction

The male testes are very sensitive and they constitute an integral part of the male reproductive system, much the same as the female ovaries. So, it's quite obvious that anything going wrong with the testes gets one anxious and on tenterhooks. Whether it's yourself or a loved one with a testicular illness, it's obviously going to be a cause of worry for the whole family. The "nuts" are, after all, single-handedly responsible for male fertility. No sperm means no babies. The testes produce your sperm, and the rest of the genital organs make sure to transport them safely to the penis for procreation. In their second equally important role, the male gonads produce testosterone, the hormone responsible for typical male attributes, such as a deep voice and muscular body.

Considering all that's at stake when one's testes are ill or diseased, it's quite normal to be concerned, or to even panic. However, most testicular illnesses are asymptomatic and aren't likely to affect your fertility or general well-being. Fortunately, they are all treatable and curable. Even the most treacherous of the testicular illnesses, testicular cancer can be cured (if detected early enough).

Most importantly, *time* is of the essence when it comes to testicular diseases. These conditions require prompt detection and immediate treatment for a positive outcome and complete cure. That does not mean one should run scared and stress over the slightest pain or the tiniest lump in the testes. Instead, it is better to educate oneself about the different aspects of the male gonads in illness and in health.

This book is a patient's guide that provides solid knowledge of the testicles. It begins with a look at the anatomy and functions of the male reproductive system, followed by the various medical conditions that most commonly affect the testes. Essential aspects such as causes, diagnosis, and prognosis are described in an easy-to-understand language for various testicular illnesses. The centerpiece for the reader is certainly the profound information on the different methods of treating and healing the testicles, including the conventional or western approach with medications and surgery, and complementary therapies like Ayurveda, Herbs, Oxygen Therapy, and Homeopathy. In order to show that even the worst of these ailments, testicular cancer, can be overcome; a section on celebrity testicular cancer survivors is included.

Once bitten, twice shy! No one likes to be affected by the same disease more than once. And so, this book provides valuable information about preventing testicular illnesses including testicular cancer. As a practical aid, a list of testicular treatment centers around the world shows you where you can go if you require the help of specialists.

Hopefully, this book answers all of your questions, and helps you take better care of yourself and your "crown jewels".

A note to the different types of readers: This book has been designed to allow quick access to information on the different testicular conditions, e.g. for those who have an actual problem and want to jump directly to the facts about it. For this purpose, please use the quick guide on page 6 as a starting point.

As a consequence of this approach, I repeat the most important information about a certain subject at the beginning of each of the "landing points" (for those who jump), so readers will understand the fundamental concepts of what is described in the following. Those among you who read this book from the first to the last page in one sitting are kindly asked to excuse the repetitions that may ensue from this approach.

All the best!

Dr. Rupert B. Hansen

1 An Overview and Quick Guide of the Book

The testes are an essential component of the male genitalia. Most importantly, they perform the vital job of making sperm and androgens, among other things. Androgens are what most people refer to as male hormones. They keep several of the bodily functions running on track, in addition to maintaining your fertility, of course. Therefore, contrary to popular opinion, the testes do much more than just produce sperm to sustain male fertility.

Sometimes, these testicular functions may begin to go wrong, or a few external factors such as bacteria or testicular trauma may send them off-track. How do you know when something like this happens within your testicles? Well, your body tells you that something's not quite right inside through its language of signs and symptoms. Unusual sensations and changes around your testicles are usually initial indicators of such illnesses. These signs can be everything from mild pain or discomfort to lumps or swelling around the testicles.

Most of these symptoms are distressing enough to raise alarming questions in your mind about your testicular health. Indeed, some of these symptoms may even sow frightening suspicions of having developed testicular cancer. Fortunately, every lump isn't necessarily cancer! As luck would have it, not even 4% of testicular lumps are tumors, out of which, only a fraction are actually malignant or cancerous [1]. Nevertheless, even the slightest pain or the tiniest lump around your testicles should be acknowledged and addressed.

Usually, young people don't expect to be affected by cancer or any such illness. However, the bad news is that testicular cancer is more of a young man's disease, with a higher incidence in 14-40-year-old males. The good news is that it's highly treatable. The most well-known example of this is Lance Armstrong, who was diagnosed with testicular cancer at the young age of 25, only to beat it over the next couple of years.

Very often, people mistake their scrotal bags for their testes. Well, the testes are actually two oval-shaped organs within the scrotal bag, so you can't see them on the outside. What you see on the outside is actually your scrotum or scrotal bag. There are several such misconceptions and incorrect information about the male genitalia floating around today. You may pick it up either on the internet or from some self-proclaimed health enthusiast, or even from some mindless locker-room repartee.

This book aims to bring clarity to the area of testicular health by busting up some of these myths and explaining what really goes on inside your body in understandable words. It's all your questions about common testicular illnesses answered in a *nutshell*.

What this book has to offer

Often, the period between noticing an unusual change around your testicles and managing to get an appointment with your doctor can be very distressing and full of anxious anticipation. You don't know what it is and you don't want to think of the myriad of ill-fated possibilities. Consequently, you go on a frantic search of the internet to end up more confused and dismayed. You don't want that! That's where this book will help ease your worries, as it aims to impart a thorough education of common testicular illnesses.

To understand any concept, you need to first get a grasp of its basics. Similarly, to understand testicular illnesses, you need to comprehend the normal structure and workings of your "balls." Because, if you know what's normal or right, only then will you know what's not right. Following this principle, this book begins with a basic explanation of the anatomy of the testes, its developmental stages through the different phases in your life, and its physiology or functions.

Next is an in-depth understanding of what can go wrong in there, which includes the more common testicular illnesses, from mere pain to cancer of the testicles. To this end, explanations on the causes, symptoms, treatments, and prognoses of these illnesses have been included, thereby acting like a systematic guide. By reading through these chapters, you will gain a well-organized picture of all these diseases in order to support you in making informed decisions on your way (back) to healthy testicles!

Most testicular illnesses are preventable. To show you how, towards the end of this book, there's a thorough guide on preventive measures to help avoid testicular illnesses, or prevent their recurrence.

Lastly, the book provides a list of several testicular health and treatment centers around the world, so you know where to go and whom to contact to find the precise solution to your specific testicular problems.

By the time you are done with this book, you will have acquired an in-depth portrait of all the aspects of testicular diseases in the simplest of languages to help you take care of your health and body.

All said and done, use it as a guide and reference book, but let a qualified physician have the last word. He/she can examine you individually and recommend appropriate measures.

Quick Guide: From Symptoms to Solutions

The following table intends to give you a brief overview of the most common symptoms of testicular health problems (left-most column) and possible conditions (columns to the right). In the two bottom rows, you will find the respective chapter and page number for a certain condition, so you can go there directly.

These symptoms...	...can be caused by the following conditions:							
	Testicular torsion	Testicular infections	Testicular cancer	Benign Testicular tumor	Spermatocele	Varicocele	Hydrocele / Haematocele	Scrotal hernia
Lump in scrotum / testes			x	x	x	x		x
Sudden sharp pain in testes	x	x						x
Dull pain in testes		x	x	x	x	x	x	x
No pain in testes /scrotum			x					
Scrotal redness	x	x					x	x
Pain in groin or lower belly	x	x	x	x	x	x	x	x
Swelling of testicles	x	x	x	x	x	x		
Please check chapter	7	6	9	8	8	8	10	9
Page no.	52	44	70	67	57	60	104, 105	99

2 Understanding the Anatomy of the Testes and Surrounding Organs

This chapter introduces you to the fundamental structure and functions of the male testicles and surrounding organs, so you can understand the terms and concepts used in the following chapters on different testicular diseases. In case you are well-versed with this part of the human body or you are eager to find out about a certain testicular illness quickly, you can jump to the chapters on the different ailments which begin on page 31.

The male genital system comprises of several components that work together, two of which being the testes enclosed within the scrotum or scrotal bag. All of these components or organs have a fixed set of functions to carry out. In the case of the testicles, it is primarily to produce the sperm and secrete testosterone. More importantly, the different organs and their respective functions are related to each other in some way and are important in maintaining your reproductive health. It is important to notice that the testes hold a crucial place in this set-up.

The testes are the male gonads, and every man usually has two of these, each located on either side of the penis (in very rare cases, doctors find three testes in the scrotum). They are also the starting point of your genitalia, in addition to being the flagship point for your sperm's journey to the finish line. The sperm travels from your testes to the Epididymis, and then through the Vas Deferens and into your Urethra and Penis. On the way, they receive a push and nourishment from the Seminal Vesicles and the Bulbourethral or Cowper's Glands located behind your urinary bladder, which do this by producing seminal fluid.

The testes begin their journey in the embryonic stage. From then until adulthood, they undergo constant development. However, some known and some unknown factors can create mild hindrances in this developmental journey of the testes. These changes often result in testicular diseases in later life. Hence, it's essential to understand the anatomy of your testes to know what's normal, before you begin to look at the possibility of an abnormality. Nevertheless, before we go on to the anatomy and development of the testes, let's have a look at the anatomy of the entire male reproductive system.

Overview of the Male Reproductive System

Humans are sexual beings, requiring the interaction of both the male as well as the female partner to procreate. The two genders are each endowed with a set of organs capable of producing specific cells for the purpose of procreation. This is where the male reproductive system or the male genitalia come in. Unlike in females, where all the reproductive organs are located inside the abdomen, most of the male reproductive organs are placed outside the body: mainly the penis, scrotum, and the testes. These organs are collectively known as the external genitalia.

The scrotum holds and protects both the testicles inside it. The reason for the external location of the testes is explained below in the section: The Descent of the Testes (page 21). Then again, there are the Seminal Vesicles, Prostate Gland, and the Vas Deferens which are located inside the body and known as the Internal Genitalia (p. 16). Let's have a look at each of these organs that constitute the reproductive system or genitalia in the males. The following image (Figure 2) shows the male genitalia and its surrounding organs, as they would appear if the body were cut into two equal parts from head to toe.

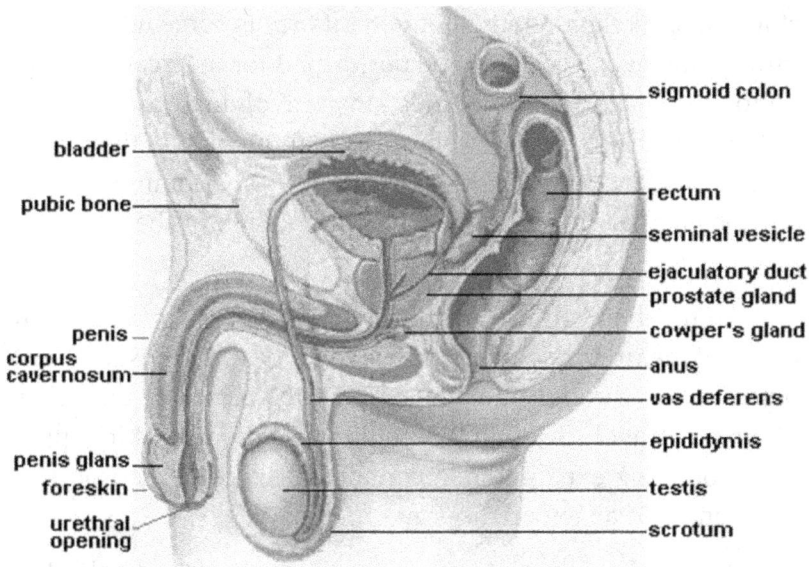

Figure 1: The Male Reproductive System
(Source: Elf Sternberg, CC BY-SA 3.0)

External Genitalia

These are organs in the male reproductive system which are placed externally or outside the abdomen.

Penis

The penis is the primary male organ with regards to sexual intercourse. It is also the most prominent of the external genitalia. It consists of three parts: namely, the root, the body or shaft, and the glans.

The root of the penis is attached to the abdominal wall and forms its anchor and base. The glans is the outer end or the cone-shaped portion of the penis. It is also known as the head of the penis. A loose fold of skin known as the prepuce covers the glans from all sides; that's the foreskin. Normally, you can move your foreskin back and forth since it's loosely attached to the penis. Sometimes, the foreskin may be absent if it has been removed in a surgical procedure known as circumcision. Circumcision is usually performed as a religious ceremony in infancy in some religions and cultures. However, it can also be performed for medical reasons in childhood or adulthood. Infections involving the foreskin, ballooning of the foreskin, or phimosis (a tightening of the foreskin that may close the opening of the penis) are some common medical conditions that are likely to require circumcision or the removal of the prepuce.

The opening that you see at the tip of the penis is actually the opening of the urethra. The urethra is the tube that transports urine and semen out through the penis. This tube begins at the urinary bladder and travels through the penis to an opening at its tip. The urethral opening expels semen containing sperm or reproductive cells when the man experiences an orgasm.

The shaft or body of the penis is cylindrical in shape and holds three circular compartments within it. Special sponge-like tissues known as the corpus spongiosum and corpus cavernosum make up one and two of these compartments, respectively. The corpus cavernosum contains the deep artery of the penis, whereas the corpus spongiosum holds the urethra. Take a look at Figure 2 to understand the placement of these tissues pictorially.

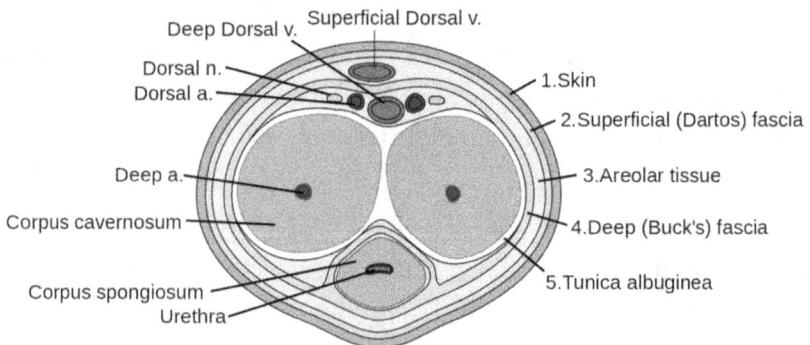

Figure 2: Cross-section of the penis
(Source: Mcstrother, CC BY 3.0)

Inside these tissues, several large spaces fill up with blood when the penis is erect during sexual arousal. This helps the penis remain rigid or erect to allow penetration for the purpose of sexual intercourse. The blood-filled tissue also helps block the urethra to avoid the passage of urine during an erection. The skin around the penile shaft is loose and elastic enough to accommodate the changes in the size of the penis during an erection.

Figure 2 above depicts the internal structure of the penis if it were to be cut at the center, horizontally. The outermost layer of the penis is the loosely attached skin followed by a layer of fat known as superficial fascia. Inside this is some more tissue and fat known as the areolar tissue and deep fascia, respectively. Finally, you have the tunica albuginea which goes on to encircle both the testes. Inside the superficial fascia or outer fat layer, you have the arteries and veins which form the major blood supply of the penis, in addition to the nerves that provide sensation. Within the tunica albuginea are two spongy compartments, corpus cavernosum which encircle the deep artery. Just below these two compartments is the single corpus spongiosum which contains the spongy urethra.

Scrotum

The scrotum is the loose pouch or sac of skin located behind the penis. This pouch holds your testes or testicles, as its primary function is to protect them from outer influences. The scrotal skin is endowed with a rich blood and nerve supply. It also contains specialized muscles that work along with another set of muscles attached to the testes known as the cremasteric muscles to act like a testicular 'climate control system.'

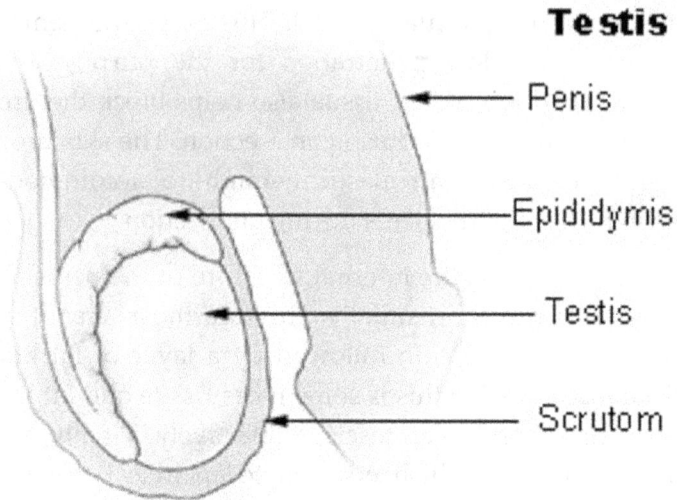

Figure 3: Scrotum and Testis

Your testes require a temperature that is 1-2 degrees lower than your core body temperature in order to produce sperm. The cremasteric muscles and the scrotum work together to maintain this optimal temperature for the testes by pulling the testes closer to the body for warmth and pushing them farther away for cooling. Learn more about this in the section "The Climate Control System of the Testes" on page 22 below.

Testes

The testes are a pair of oval-shaped organs situated in the loose pouches of the scrotum. They are also referred to as the male gonads. Under normal circumstances, every male has two testes that are housed in the scrotal bag behind the penis. A septum (wall of tissue) divides the scrotum in two pouches and keeps the testes separated from each other. The testicles are located obliquely in the scrotal pouches, with the left one usually sitting a little lower than the right one. The spermatic cord from above and the scrotal ligament from below keep the testes moored to the scrotum. The tunica vaginalis testis (a serous covering) engulfs the testes from the outside in two layers. Below this layer is the tough fibrous outer covering of the testes, the tunica albuginea. A comma-shaped structure known as the epididymis, which is a highly convoluted and tightly packed tube, is attached to the posterior end of the testicles (see Figure 5, page 10).

Each of the ovoid testes typically measures 3.5-5 cm (1.38-1.9 inches) long, 2.5-3 cm (0.98-1.1 inches) wide, and 3 cm (1.1 inches) deep, with a volume of 25 ml (0.8 oz.). On the outside, the testes have a smooth texture. Picture a small plum or large olive, and you'll get an idea of how an adult testis looks from the outside (see Figure 4).

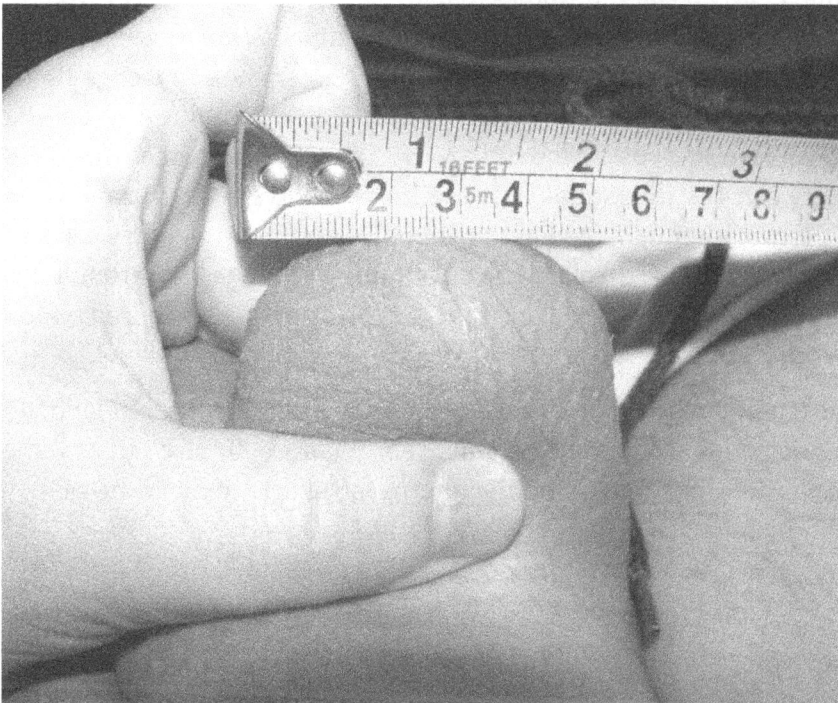

Figure 4: Size of an adult male's testicle
(Source: Richie, CC BY-SA3.0)

The testes undergo a growth spurt at puberty in response to the advent of spermatogenesis, which means production of sperm. The amount of sperm produced, interstitial fluid, and the number of sertoli cells all determine the size of your "balls". Generally, the volume of each testis in adulthood is likely to be around 500% more than their pre-pubertal volume.

Internally, the testes are made up of several lobules. Within these lobules are several tubes or glandular tubules held together by loose connective tissues. These small tubes are known as the seminiferous tubules and they are responsible for producing your sperm. There are about 700 such tubules in each testicle. The seminiferous tubules are scattered with sperm in various stages of development. These canals come together at the center to merge into nearly 30 larger tubules that again merge into 15 larger straight tubules. The latter pierce the tunica albuginea (fibrous covering of the testis) and go on to form the epididymis. The connective tissue is also interspersed with interstitial cells containing the Leydig cells. These cells are where your testosterone comes from. In between the interstitial cells are the Sertoli cells that provide the sperm with much-needed nutrition. Due to their role, they are also known as 'nurse cells'. If you would slice a testis through the middle along its long axis, it is likely to appear like a sliced lemon from the inside due to the many lobes and tubes it contains.

The following Figure 5 shows the location of the testis in relation to the scrotal pouch, penis, and epididymis. It also shows the seminiferous tubules and the internal structure of the testicles.

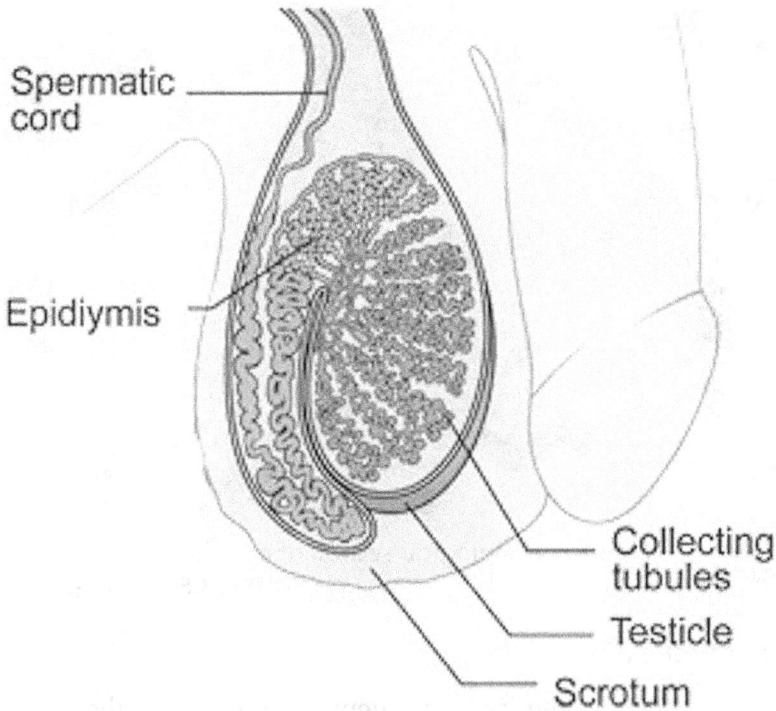

Figure 5: Inner structure of the testes
(Source: Cancer Research UK, CC BY-SA 4.0)

The next picture (Figure 6) shows how the testes appear under the high-power lens of a microscope. The circular structures are the seminiferous tubules with a central lumen. What you see in between them is the connective tissue with the leydig and sertoli cells. The dark spots within the larger round structures are sperm in different stages of development.

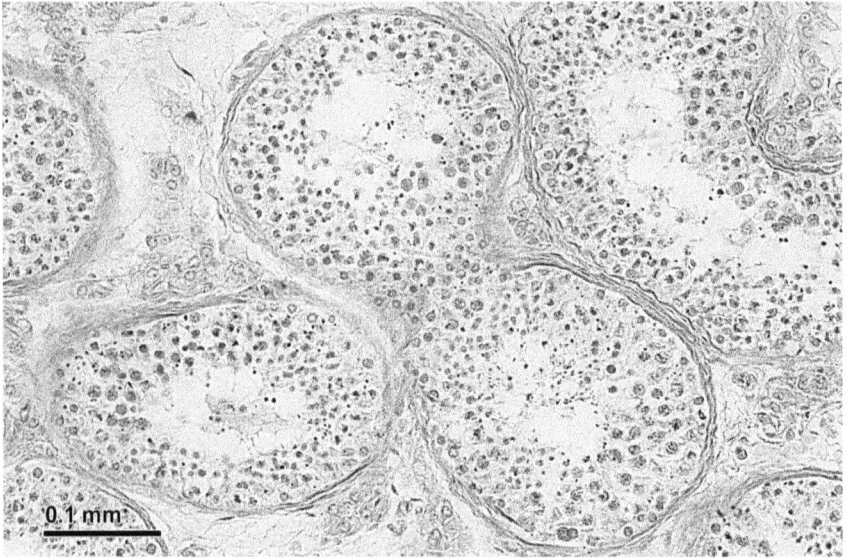

Figure 6: Histological section of a testis
(Source: Dr. Josef Reischig, CSc., CC BY-SA 3.0)

Internal Genitalia

This brings us to the internal genital organs of the male reproductive system. These organs are sometimes referred to as the accessory organs, too.

Epididymis

This is a long, highly convoluted, and tightly coiled tube resting at the back of each testis. It is attached to the posterior-end of the testis, and its job is to store the sperm while they mature and subsequently transport the mature sperm to the Vas Deferens. It's that coma-shaped tube you see behind the testes (see Figure 7 below). It is actually a 20-foot long tube tightly coiled to fit into a small space. This long length serves the sperm with a storage area and enough time to reach maturity.

It consists of three parts: the head or the caput epididymis, the body, and the tail or cauda.

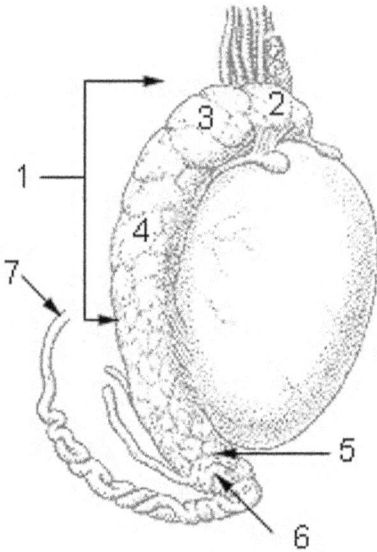

1. Epididymis
2. Caput Epididymis
3. Lobules of Epididymis
4. Body of Epididymis
5. Tail of Epididymis
6. Duct of Epididymis
7. Vas Deferens

Figure 7: Testis and Epididymis

The sperm that come out of the testis are immature and inept for fertilization. From the testicles, the immature sperm first enter the caput epididymis and travel through the body of the epididymis to enter its cauda or tail. They remain here until they have reached maturity, thus becoming capable of bringing about fertilization. Usually, each sperm remains in the epididymis for 2-3 months before it enters the Vas Deferens. The contractions around the penis during sexual arousal force the sperm into this connecting tube. From the Vas Deferens, they travel to the urethra and then outside the urethral opening at the tip of the penis.

Vas Deferens

The Vas Deferens is a long, muscular tube that begins at tail of the epididymis and travels through the pelvic cavity to open into the urethra just behind the urinary bladder (refer Figure 1, page 9). It transports mature sperm from the tail of the epididymis to the urethra, a tube in which they travel through the penis towards the penile tip. During sexual arousal, the Vas Deferens undergoes muscular movements known as peristalsis to transport the sperm for ejaculation. Peristalsis is a series of muscular contractions and relaxations along a tube to produce a wave-like movement. This movement helps push the contents of the tube forward.

Seminal Vesicles

These organs are a pair of sac-like structures attached to the Vas Deferens behind the urinary bladder (see Figure 8, page 19). The seminal vesicles produce a fluid that provides the sperm with nourishment and the energy to move forward. This fluid is rich in sugar, mainly fructose, which is essential for the movement of the sperm. The seminal fluid makes up most of a man's ejaculate.

Ejaculatory Ducts

The Vas Deferens and the seminal vesicles fuse to form the ejaculatory ducts. These ducts open and empty the ejaculate into the urethra.

Urethra

In males, the urethra is a tube that extends from the opening of the urinary bladder to the tip of the penis. Its primary function is to drain and eliminate the urine from the bladder. However, in males, it has an additional function of transporting the ejaculate and sperm out of the penis at the time of orgasm. During sexual intercourse, the erect penis blocks the flow of urine to allow only the semen to ejaculate out of the urethra.

Prostate Gland

The prostate gland is situated just below the urinary bladder and in front of the rectum. It is a donut-shaped gland that sits around the urethra. So, the urethra actually runs through the center of this gland. A healthy prostate gland is about the size of a walnut. This gland produces the so-called prostatic fluid responsible for providing nourishment to the sperm.

The following picture (Figure 8) shows the location of the prostate gland in relation to the bladder, rectum, and urethra.

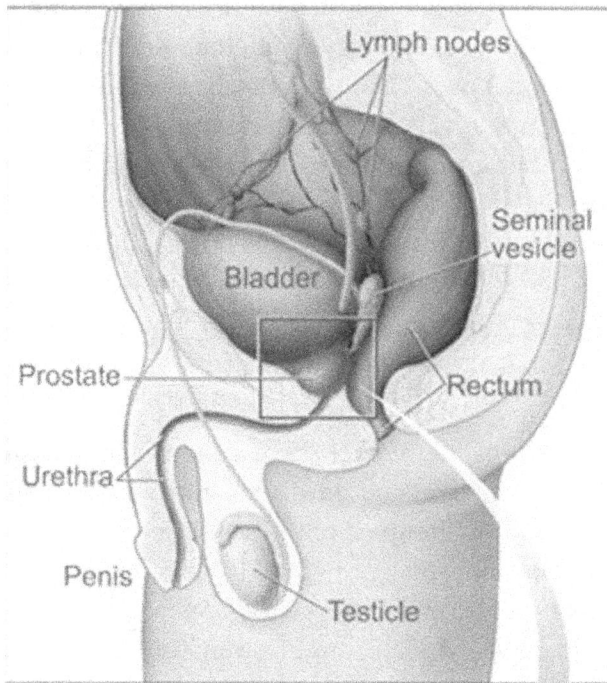

This shows the prostate and nearby organs.

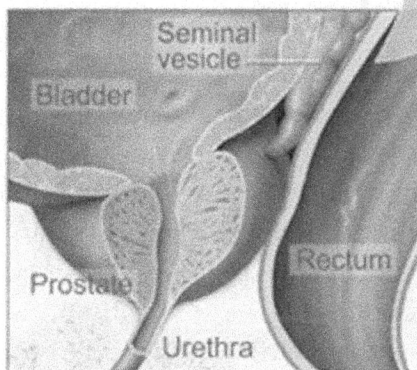

This shows the inside of the prostate, urethra, rectum, and bladder.

Figure 8: The Prostate gland in relation to its adjacent organs

Bulbourethral or Cowper's Glands

These glands are small, pea-sized organs situated just below the prostate gland on both sides of the urethra (Refer Figure 1, page 9). They secrete clear and slippery fluid that lubricates the urethra during sexual intercourse. It also neutralizes any acidity along the urethra which may result from residual drops of urine left behind in the urethra before the urinary flow is cut-off during a penile erection. An acidic atmosphere in the urethra is prone to damaging the sperm, and so this fluid neutralizes this acidity.

The growth of the testes in the womb and through infancy

The development of the reproductive system is mainly a prenatal process. Since it involves the development of the sex organs, this process is also an integral part of the sex differentiation process in the embryo. The embryonic growth of these organs is an important aspect of fetal development because any abnormalities in this process could have possible ramifications on future fertility and sexual health. Not surprisingly, lately researchers are increasingly realizing the fact that we may find answers to most medical questions if the fetal development was studied more closely.

The testes and the rest of the male reproductive organs develop from the so-called intermediate mesoderm. The permanent reproductive organs of the adult male are preceded by the Wolffian ducts or mesonephric ducts that are purely embryonic in nature. This structure looks like a duct or tunnel within the womb of the growing embryo. The male reproductive system gradually begins to form from these ducts. The ducts disappear almost entirely before the fetal life ends at birth. Similarly, the Mullerian ducts form the female reproductive organs in women. However, these ducts are also present in the male embryo but they reduce in size and become inactive, as the Wolffian ducts take over the formation of the male reproductive organs, once your embryo executes the chromosomal information to become a male.

The embryo consists of three basic layers, the outer layer or the ectoderm, the middle layer or the mesoderm, and the inner layer or the endoderm. Each of these layers plays an important role in the development of the fetus or baby. The various organs in your body, from your hair and skin to your bones have developed from these layers. The outer region of the intermediate mesoderm in the embryo forms the Wolffian duct. This embryonic canal forms the tube of the epididymis that transfers sperm from the testes to the Vas Deferens. The seminal vesicles arise from this duct around the third month of fetal life. They are located behind the urinary bladder and are responsible for producing seminal fluid that forms part of the semen and provides nourishment to the sperm. Before the Wolffian ducts disappear, they also form a part of the testicles or their efferent ducts. The rest of the gonads or the testes develop from the mesothelium layer of the peritoneum.

The tunica albuginea develops as the outer layer of the testes. This is followed by the development of rete testis, a central network of cords. Another network develops the seminiferous tubules that are connected to the efferent ducts of the testes [2], [3].

The Descent of the Testes

This is an important phenomenon in the fetal phase of the developing testes. The testes are located in the anterior abdominal wall of the fetus as they develop and grow. Around week 10-15 of gestation, while the baby continues to grow within the mother's womb, the testes begin to move down slowly to their final position within the scrotal pouches. The opening of a tunnel-like connection from the testes in the abdominal wall to the scrotal pouches heralds this descent. Simultaneously, the gubernaculum, a muscle attached to the testes begins to develop. The gubernaculum pulls the testes into the developing scrotal bags on both sides. Normally, once the testes have descended these passages fuse and close behind them. Unfortunately in some men, these passages fail to do so. Such a failure to close down increases the chances of an indirect scrotal/inguinal hernia (see page 99) or infantile hydrocele (see page 104).

97% of full term babies and 70% of preterm babies are born with both testes that have already descended into the scrotal pouches. Among those that are born with undescended testes, usually just one of the testicles remains undescended and even that one is likely to descend sometime in the baby's first year.

Of course, there are instances when the testes do not descend into the scrotal bags at all. Such a condition is known as cryptorchidism or ectopic testis. Most of the time, such anomalies can be corrected with surgery [4].

So, why is it important for the testes to descend down into the externally placed scrotal pouches? There is a vital reason for this relocation. Your testes require a temperature few degrees lower than your core body temperature to be able to produce sperm. Hence, once they have developed they descend down into the scrotal out-pockets or pouches. In here, the temperature is 1-2 degrees lower than your core body temperature, which is optimal for the manufacture of the sperm and the maintenance of sperm quality.

The Climate Control System of the Testes

The cremasteric muscles in the scrotum are capable of contracting and relaxing to adjust the position of the testes. They contract and pull the testes closer to the body during cold weather or as a protective response during a fight. They are bound to relax again when the testes require a cooler atmosphere. This phenomenon is known as the cremasteric reflex. It helps to keep your testes protected and in a constant sperm-generation mode like a well-oiled machine. The cremasteric reflex can also be visualized by stroking the inner thigh just below the scrotum. The stroking is likely to pull the testicles upwards as the cremasteric muscles contract to pull them closer to the body.

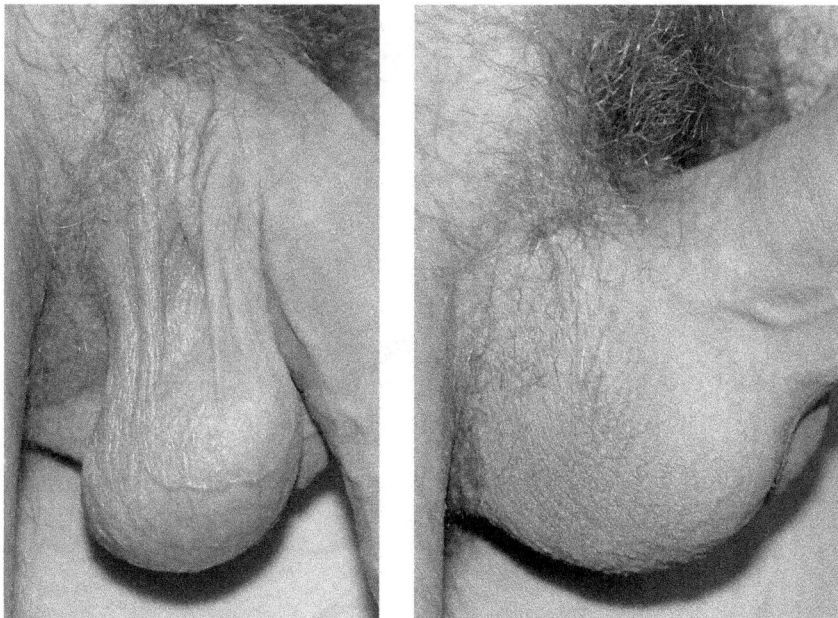

Figure 9: Scrotum in relaxed and tense state
(Source: 123GLGL, CC BY-SA 3.0)

3   What are the Testes Designed to do?

The testes or male gonads are the male sex glands, similar to the ovaries in women. The purpose of your testes is mainly two-fold: to produce sperm, and release the male hormone, testosterone. Although, the production of sperm is important for your virility, the androgens secreted by the testes are vital for the regulation of various bodily functions and for your masculinity. Yes, the facial hair, thick voice, and other manly traits are attributed to the presence of this hormone. So much so that, testosterone is what keeps your sex drive going too.

Let's focus in on these two important functions of the testes.

Spermatogenesis

Spermatogenesis is the medical term for the production of sperm within the testes. This process occurs in the sertoli cells, located inside the seminiferous tubules (see Figure 6, page 16). The spermatozoa are produced from the male primordial germ cells through the processes of mitosis and meiosis.

The very first cells to begin this process are the spermatogonia that form primary spermatocytes through mitosis (cell division). These primary spermatocytes then divide by "meiosis I" to form two secondary spermatocytes (Figure 10). Each of these secondary spermatocytes divides into two spermatids through "meiosis II" to finally develop into mature spermatozoa or sperm. In this manner, each spermatogonia cell ends up producing four sperm in the end [5].

The following picture (Figure 11) shows how the sperm are arranged inside the testicles during their developmental phase.

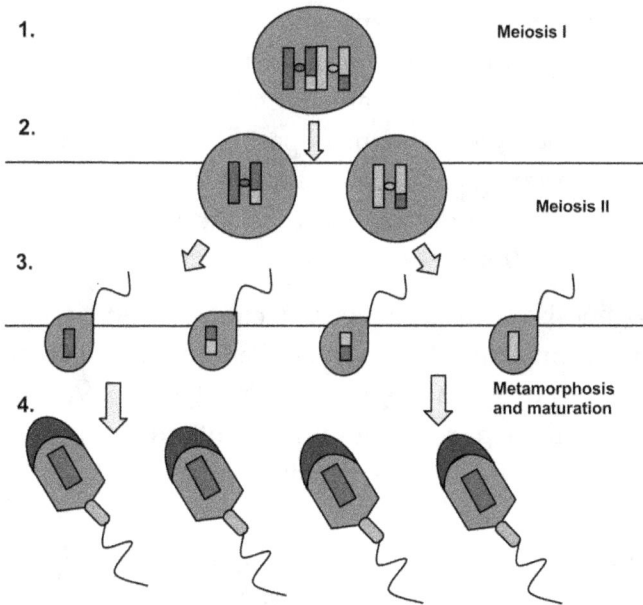

Figure 10: Four stages of spermatogenesis
(Source: Anchor207, CC BY-SA 3.0)

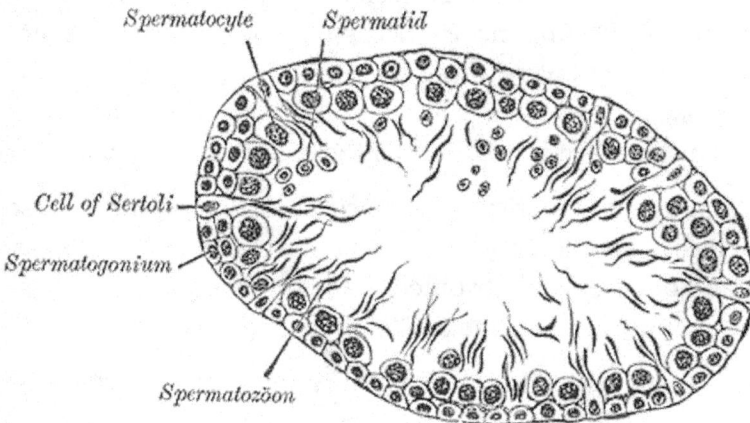

Figure 11: Spermatogenesis in the Testis
(Source: Henry Gray)

The sperm then travel from the seminiferous tubules into the epididymis (see Figure 5). It's here that they reach maturity to finally enter the Vas Deferens and mix with the seminal and prostatic fluids on their way out of the urethra. The whole process of sperm formation and maturity takes about 7 weeks. The interaction of the hypothalamus (a part of the brain), the pituitary gland (an important gland located at the base of the brain), and the hormones produced by the sertoli cells and the leydig cells in the testes essentially stimulates and regulates this process.

Spermatogenesis begins at puberty to continue until death. In fact, at any given time, an adult man is likely to have several cells in different stages of spermatogenesis in his testicles. Although this process once initiated, continues until death, the number of sperm produced is likely to reduce gradually with age.

Testosterone

The leydig cells interspersed within the connective tissues in the testes are the primary source of the male hormone, testosterone. As a result, your testes are majorly responsible for the testosterone levels in your blood stream. Testosterone is an extremely vital male sex hormone. Its presence is necessary for the development of certain manly traits and reproductive functions. The secretion of testosterone by the leydig cells also keeps the production of sperm going. This means it is required for the maintenance of fertility too.

Typical male characteristics like facial hair, body hair, hoarse or deep voice, wide shoulders, increased muscle and bone mass, body odor, and oily skin are attributed to the presence of testosterone. It also maintains the sex drive and stamina in males.

A testosterone deficiency is likely to result in fatigue, depression, osteoporosis, and a low sex drive in a man. Some men may also experience hot flushes due to a low testosterone level. Yes, hot flushes aren't only a female thing; they can most certainly occur in males too.

For instance, *eunuchs* have much lower levels of testosterone in their blood than normal males, which is the main reason why they lack most of the secondary sexual characteristics. The Mosby's Medical Dictionary describes a eunuch as a man whose testicles are either damaged or have been removed. No testicles means no or miniscule testosterone in the blood. No testosterone means a lack of or abnormal secondary sexual characteristics. That's why most eunuchs tend to have a feminine voice and lack of facial hair.

Just the same, testosterone levels in childhood are much lower than in adulthood because the testes mainly begin to function at puberty. Until then, the testes are still in the developmental stages, reaching maturity when a boy reaches puberty. So, puberty is when the testes begin to produce testosterone in the true sense. Hence, it is at this juncture that a boy suddenly develops a hoarse, cracking voice and facial hair. Some boys also experience an outbreak of acne at puberty as a result of increasingly oily skin from increased testosterone levels. The following picture (Figure 12) portrays the development of androgenic hair or male patterns of body hair according to age.

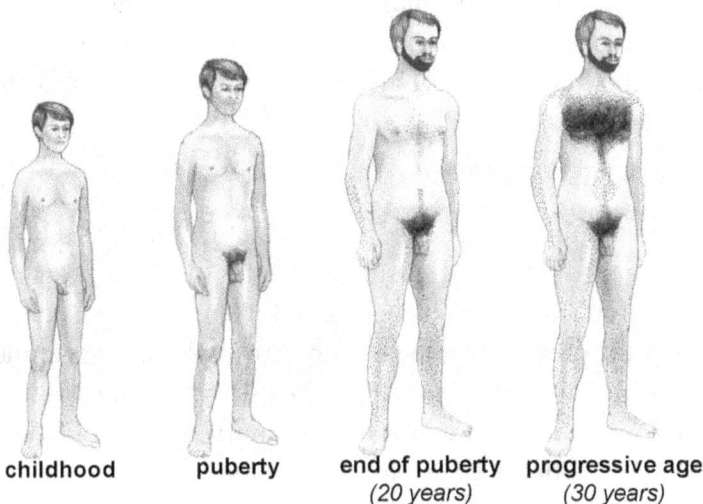

childhood   puberty   end of puberty   progressive age
(20 years)   *(30 years)*

Figure 12: Androgenic hair patterns due to testosterone

(Source: IGenesis89, CC BY-SA 3.0)

4   What happens when things begin to go wrong?

Generally, we take many things around us for granted, including our health and bodies. Take for instance your heart, which on an average beats 72 times every minute. Do you feel or hear it beating inside your chest? Normally, most of us would answer this question with a 'NO.' Since, more often than not, you are oblivious to your heart's constant beating and pumping.

Although you do not feel it pump, it's still transporting blood to every tiny corner of your body. When you experience a scare or are exposed to a situation of extreme anxiety, then your heart begins to beat faster and you can feel it pump inside your chest cavity. This is known as palpitation. Thus, unless something goes wrong you aren't likely to notice your heart doing its daily chores.

Most of us treat our overall health and bodies in this manner. We remember to eat and keep it clean, but that's about it. Your body carries out a myriad of functions, some big and some small, on a daily basis. Usually, you hardly feel anything when everything's fine or working in harmony. However, the moment something goes amiss, you are likely to feel anything from mere tiredness to pain. That's DISEASE.

DISEASE = DIS + EASE

Disease is the absence of ease or well-being. All of this holds true for your reproductive and testicular health too. Testicular health is of paramount importance, especially for the maintenance of male fertility. Normally, your testes produce male sex hormones and sperm daily like clockwork. Nonetheless, the moment something goes wrong, things are apt to go awry with your testicular functions. So, what happens in such a situation?

A diseased testis starts sending out SOS signals in the form of lumps, pain, or inflammation. Some of these symptoms require immediate attention, whereas others may just go away by themselves with time. Sadly, there's no way to know the severity of your symptoms without investigating their cause.

The most basic symptom of any disease is discomfort or pain. In the case of your testes, pain could indicate everything from a slight injury during a routine workout to testicular torsion. Testicular torsion (chapter 7, page 52) is by far the most critical medical condition of the testicles after testicular cancer. It comes with severe pain and requires immediate medical intervention to prevent the loss of testicular functions on the affected side. Nevertheless, other conditions like testicular infections, benign testicular lumps, and scrotal conditions and hernias can cause pain around your testes, too.

After pain, the other symptom that one would probably notice in the testicular area is lumps or swelling (chapter 8, page 57). A lump anywhere in the body, whether painful or not, often sends alarm bells ringing in even the calmest of minds. You need not necessarily be a hypochondriac to connect a lump with cancer. Even so, not all lumps are cancer. Moreover, in the case of testicular lumps, a mere 4% of these are classified as tumors, of which even fewer are actually cancerous [1]. So, what else could a testicular lump indicate? Well, it could be a Varicocele (enlarged vein, see page 60) or a Testicular cyst/ Spermatocele (fluid and sperm-filled cyst, page 57).

Then again, there are disorders of the scrotal pouches that could be mistaken for testicular infirmities. These scrotal diseases such as unchecked Hydrocele (page 104) or Scrotal/ Inguinal hernias (page 99) may sometimes harm the testicles too. Thus, there's a lot that could go wrong around your nuts.

Fortunately, with the advanced investigations and detection techniques available today, finding out what's wrong with your testes is nearly always possible. Furthermore, state of the art surgical techniques and other treatment methods enable correction of these testicular problems in the vast majority of cases.

This book discusses all of the aforementioned testicular illnesses in detail in the subsequent chapters.

5 Testicular Pain: An Alarm Signal to be Checked

Testicular pain can send quite a few men in a tizzy. It's there, you take note, and the next moment it's gone, only to be back again after a while. Not knowing what's going on inside your gonads and wondering why they hurt can leave you feeling anxious and stressed for your well-being. Then again, locker room stories of testicular pain turning out to be something more serious may add more fuel to the fire, and keep you on tenterhooks until you know what it is.

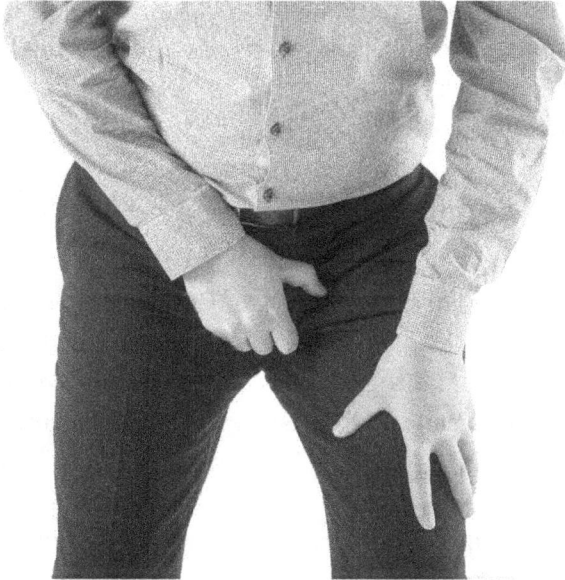

Fortunately, most cases of testicular pain aren't as serious as they may appear. In fact, most of these instances of pain get better with medication and precautionary measures alone. But, until you know what stands behind your testicular pain, you are bound to worry and speculate. Instead of worrying yourself into a fit, you have the option of learning about testicular pain. This chapter aims to decode such individual pains in their different aspects to help you understand your testicular aches better and act accordingly.

Symptoms

Testicular pain is a symptom in itself and not a separate medical condition. It usually points towards some underlying testicular disease. Aching in the testes typically varies in type, intensity, and nature depending on the underlying cause. Seen from a statistical point of view, testicular pain is not too common, as only approximately 1 in 4000 men under 25 years of age experience it [6].

When you complain of testicular pain to your healthcare provider, the first thing he/she would do is to rule out severe and sudden pain from testicular torsion. Testicular torsion is the most serious cause of pain in the testicles which requires immediate medical attention. A torsion of the spermatic cord and the muscles holding the testes cuts off the blood flow to the testes, leading to irreversible harm in a relatively short time. Hence, you can't afford to ignore severe testicular pain, as there's a chance that it's due to testicular torsion. Read more about this condition in chapter 7, page 52.

Before you go off thinking that your testicular pain could be due to testicular torsion, hold your horses. Of course, if your pain is sudden and severe, there's a high chance it's torsion, but there are certain other medical conditions that could also result in strong testicular pain. Testicular infection or Orchitis, and Epididymitis are some of these alternate causes. To differentiate from torsions, such conditions are more prone to causing testicular pain that comes gradually and increases slowly. Additionally, testicular pain localized to a particular area also suggests a testicular infection or epididymitis.

The cause of one's testicular pain can be narrowed down by evaluating the symptoms accompanying it. Here's a list of some accessory symptoms that usually accompany testicular pain from various causes (more on the possible causes on the following pages):

- Testicular or scrotal swelling, tenderness, and/or redness, along with pain. Such symptoms more often indicate a testicular infection
- Fever with testicular pain also signifies an underlying infection
- Painful urination or penile discharge with testicular pain
- Pain during sexual intercourse or ejaculation
- Nausea and vomiting frequently accompanies testicular pain in testicular torsion
- Blood in urine or semen

Whatever may be the cause or nature of testicular pain, the first and the most important step is always to rule out testicular torsion. This one condition should never be ignored, as it's a true medical emergency.

Here's a table to help differentiate between the pain from testicular torsion and other causes:

Testicular torsion	Other testicular pain
Sudden onset of pain	Gradual onset of pain
Severe, unbearable pain	Severe pain
Pain is located around the testes, scrotum, and abdomen	Pain may be localized to a single region of the scrotum
Continuous pain	Pain may come and go
Nausea and vomiting	No nausea and vomiting
Unusually positioned testicles, higher than normal	Normally positioned testicles

Causes

Testicular pain can crop up from a variety of possible causes. Some of these call for immediate medical measures, whereas others aren't as serious as they may appear. However, it's best to treat every case of severe testicular pain as a medical emergency until all the grave possibilities have been ruled out. The following is a list of all the potential causes of testicular pain.

Epididymitis

Epididymitis is the inflammation of the epididymis at the posterior end of the testis (see Figure 7, page 17). This is the most common cause of testicular pain in men above 18 years of age. Generally, sexually active men are liable to contract epididymitis as a result of STDs (Sexually Transmitted Diseases) like gonorrhea and chlamydia, whereas elderly men are more likely to get it due to an enlarged prostate gland.

Trauma

Trauma to the testes is a regular cause of extreme testicular pain. Such pain from a direct injury to the scrotum is often excruciating, but it also tends to be only temporary. Nearly 85% of the testicular injuries are from blunt trauma as from a kick or punch to the scrotum, sports injuries, straddle injuries, or car accidents. Most of the time, such trauma causes bruises and swelling around the scrotum.

Testicular torsion

Testicular torsion (see page 52) is the twisting of a testicle inside the scrotum. The spermatic cord that holds the testicle in position also contains the artery and vein supplying blood to the testis within it. As a result, when a testicle twists along the spermatic cord, the twisting is likely to cut-off its blood supply too, resulting in a medical emergency. The subsequent effect of testicular torsion is severe and sudden pain in the abdomen and scrotal pouches with nausea and vomiting.

Testicular inflammation or orchitis

Inflammation of the testes or Orchitis is another cause of testicular pain. Orchitis is usually a fall-out of the mumps virus in young boys. However, it can also result from an untreated epididymitis in an adult male. Even so, several other viral and bacterial strains are also known to cause this type of infection (more on this on page 44 and following).

Testicular tumors

Testicular tumors rarely cause pain in the testicles, as most tumors are painless, especially the malignant or cancerous ones (see chapter 8, page 57). However, tumors may cause pain under certain circumstances, particularly when they exert pressure on the surrounding organs or nerves.

Inguinal hernia

Scrotal/ Inguinal hernias sometimes lead to testicular pain or discomfort with scrotal swelling. This condition is the protrusion of the intestines into the scrotal pouch through a muscular defect in the abdominal wall (see also chapter 1, page 99).

Kidney stones

Kidney stones do not usually cause pain in the testes, but occasionally, such pain may radiate down to the testes too.

Vasectomy

A vasectomy in the past, at times, causes mild to severe pain in the testicles. This is known as 'Post-vasectomy Pain Syndrome.' The condition affects every 1 in 3 vasectomized males.

A vasectomy is a surgical intervention conducted to sterilize a man by interrupting and sealing his Vas Deferens (see page 17) on both the left and right side. Accordingly, the sperm can no longer enter the ejaculate, and thereby fertilization of female eggs becomes impossible. A vasectomy may cause testicular pain immediately or after a while, even after several years. The pain can range from mild to debilitating, and can be intermittent or permanent. It may arise during an erection or sexual intercourse, which is especially disturbing. A vasectomy seals or blocks the transport of the sperm from the Epididymis into the ejaculate, but it doesn't stop the production of sperm. This unstopped production of the sperm in the testicles leads to a back-pressure built-up in the epididymis, which in turn might cause post-vasectomy testicular pain. Another reason is the possibility of nerve damage around the epididymis during the vasectomy procedure and due to the subsequent development of fibrous tissue or scars around the region of the vasectomy.

Diagnosis

A healthcare professional diagnoses the underlying cause of testicular pain by conducting a complete physical examination with diagnostic tests and an in-depth history of the complaints.

Physical examination:

The physical examination of a patient with testicular pain mainly focuses on the abdomen, groin, scrotum, testes, and penis. The healthcare professional palpates or feels the abdomen and scrotum to look for swelling, lumps, tenderness, and discolorations. Normally, a scrotal swelling with pain would rule out testicular involvement. Such a swelling is more likely a Hydrocele or Scrotal/ Inguinal hernia.

Laboratory tests and Imaging:

Your healthcare professional may suggest the following examinations to help diagnose the cause of your testicular pain:

- **Complete Blood Count** to check for the levels of white blood cells and other infection parameters.
- **Urine analysis** to check for blood and bacteria in the urine.
- **Urethral swab** to look for sexually transmitted diseases in case of penile discharge.

- **Testicular Ultrasound**, a non-invasive imaging technique that creates a visual image of the blood flow to the testes for diagnosing testicular torsion. This test also helps detect anatomical abnormalities in the scrotum and testes like hematoceles, abscesses, testicular ruptures, testicular tumors, and inguinal hernias. In addition, a testicular ultrasound is also likely to detect epididymitis or orchitis. Since inflammation increases the blood flow to the affected areas, a testicular ultrasound can detect it by evaluating the blood flow in and around the suspected areas.
- **Nuclear scan** is performed by injecting a radioactive dye through an IV line. This test looks for abnormalities in the blood flow of the testes. Areas wherein the blood flow is affected show a decreased collection of dye. For instance, testicular torsion (see page 52) shows reduced uptake of dye in the affected testis during a scan, as torsion cuts off the testicular blood flow.

These investigations are useful in diagnosing most or all of the causes of testicular pain. However, testicular torsion does not leave much time for lengthy investigations. That's why, on occasions where a high suspicion of testicular torsion exists, healthcare professionals begin preparation for surgery immediately without wasting valuable time on investigations to salvage the affected testicle.

Treating Testicular Pain

Conventional treatment

The treatment of testicular pain depends on its underlying cause. The most urgent of its causes, testicular torsion, is treated with emergency surgery. The faster such a testis is operated on, the better are the chances of saving it. Testicular torsion surgery realigns the testis by detangling the twist along the spermatic cord to restore the blood supply to the affected testicle. We will be discussing testicular torsion in more detail in chapter 7, page 52.

Testicular pain in general is treated with pain medications, ice packs, rest, and scrotal support with athletic scrotal supporters or jockstraps. Furthermore, an underlying inflammation or infection would also call for specific antibiotics against the bacteria responsible for the infection and testicular pain. Inguinal hernia or hydrocele necessitates surgery in addition to pain medications, scrotal support, and rest. Testicular tumors, especially if malignant, entail surgery for the removal of the affected testicle.

Let's look at the treatment options for each of the causes of testicular pain separately.

Trauma:

Treatment for testicular trauma includes the following after careful evaluation of the underlying testicular injury.

- Pain and anti-inflammatory medications
- Scrotal elevation with support
- Ice packs
- Rest

Testicular surgery may be required after severe trauma to the testes that may have caused a hematocele or a collection of blood in the scrotum, testicular rupture, or penetrating injuries.

Testicular torsion:

Testicular torsion needs nothing but immediate surgery. A urologist may attempt manual untwisting of the testes to relieve the torsion before attempting surgery. Surgical measures for testicular torsion include untwisting of the affected testis, assessment of its viability, and securing the testis to the scrotal wall through so-called orchiopexy. This securing of the testis prevents subsequent testicular torsion in the future. Most of the time, the urologist secures the other unaffected testes to the scrotal wall too as a preventive measure against future torsion episodes.

Epididymitis and orchitis:

Epididymitis and orchitis are typically treated with the following measures:

- 10-14 days of antibiotic therapy. The choice of antibiotic depends on the type of infection and age of the patient.
- Pain and anti-inflammatory medications
- Scrotal elevation and support
- Ice packs to relieve pain and inflammation
- Rest

Testicular tumors:

Testicular tumors require prompt evaluation by a urologist to diagnose the type of tumor. Once diagnosed, testicular cancers are treated with a combination of chemotherapy, radiation, and surgery. We will discuss these treatment options in more detail in chapter 9, which starts on page 70.

Inguinal hernia:

Inguinal hernias require surgery to push the protruding intestines back into the abdominal cavity. Individuals with hernias are frequently advised to refrain from straining and lifting heavy weights (more in chapter 1, page 99).

Kidney stone:

Although this is a rare cause of testicular pain, it is still a possibility. Kidney stones are treated with pain medications and diuretics like tamsulosin. These drugs aim to flush out the stone(s) by increasing the frequency of urination. Sometimes, a kidney stone may need surgery depending on its size.

Alternative Therapy

Natural therapies are also likely to help with testicular pain. However, it's always better to get your pain diagnosed by a healthcare professional before you turn to these therapies for pain relief. You want to get yourself diagnosed mainly because the efficacy of each herb often changes as per its underlying medical cause. More importantly, medical emergencies like testicular torsion, trauma, and testicular cancer necessitate immediate surgical measures. Hence, trying alternative measures instead of surgery bears the danger of just making such diseases worse. The rest of the causes of testicular pain are often treated successfully with the correct alternative measures. Let's see how.

Ayurveda and herbs

Ayurveda is an effective option for testicular pain from epididymitis or orchitis. This type of pain and also testicular swelling is said to get better with the following ayurvedic herbal preparations. Most of the ingredients in these preparations are available in herbal stores and on the internet. Make sure you check the authenticity and quality of these products before you use them.

- Mix equal parts of Kanuga or Indian Beech seeds, castor seeds, and bonduc plant seeds. Grind with castor oil to make a thick paste. Apply this paste on the groin or swollen area overnight. Wash it off the next morning. Ideally, you are supposed to apply this paste every night until the swelling subsides.
- Grind a few pomegranate leaves to make a paste. Application of this paste over the scrotum is likely to reduce testicular pain and discomfort.
- Boil a few pieces of raw papaya and grind to make a paste. Application of this paste over the scrotum or groin can reduce swelling.

You may use any one of the above herbal preparations at a time, to ease testicular pain. In case you have any underlying medical conditions, speak to your doctor before trying herbal remedies to rule out drug interactions and side effects. It is recommended that you consult an ayurvedic physician to find out the best herbal remedies for your pain.

Homeopathy

Homeopathy is a safe and effective therapeutic option for many of the common testicular complaints. Testicular pain on the right side or testicular conditions affecting the right testis often gets better with Staphysagria. Epididymitis or orchitis infections due to organisms that cause gonorrhea are known to get better with Pulsatilla or Clematis. Shooting, dragging, and pulling pain in the groin and thighs would indicate Pulsatilla, whereas a hard testicle accompanied by increased pain at night and from cold would indicate Clematis. Extreme soreness of the testicles is treated with Hamamelis.

We will discuss the treatment options for each of these specific testicular conditions in more detail in the following chapters.

Prognosis

The prognosis of testicular pain is entirely dependent on the underlying cause that leads up to the pain.

The outcome of testicular pain from trauma depends on the extent and severity of the injury. Most patients with mild to moderate testicular trauma are expected to recover without any long-term effects, but others with severe trauma may suffer permanent damage and loss of a testicle.

The prognosis of testicular torsion depends on the time elapsed from the onset of the symptoms to the successful de-torsion of the testis, manually or surgically. The chances of saving the testis reduce drastically with time.

Time elapsed between symptom onset to de-torsion	Rate of salvaging the testis
Within 6 hours	90-100%
After 12 hours	20-50%
After 24 hours	0-10%

The complications involved with testicular torsion are loss of the affected testis, permanently damaged testis, infertility, and/or infection.

A testicular pain prognosis for epididymitis or orchitis is quite good. Most of the individuals who undergo appropriate antibiotic therapy for these conditions recover without any complications. On the contrary, if left untreated, these infections tend to cause abscesses, altered fertility, and sometimes sepsis wherein the infection spreads through the blood to other more important organs. Therefore, timely medication for epididymitis and orchitis is essential.

The prognosis of testicular tumors depends on the type and extent of the tumor at the time of its diagnosis.

As for inguinal hernias (see page 99), the prognosis is good if surgical correction of the hernia is performed before it gets obstructed. An obstructed or irreversible inguinal hernia may lead to loss of the intestinal segment trapped in the groin or scrotal pouch. However, most cases of inguinal hernias improve after surgery. The surgeon also usually places a mesh along the abdominal wall to provide it with additional support and to help avoid the recurrence of an inguinal hernia in the future.

Quick summary of testicular pain

Condition	Testicular Pain
Main symptoms	Severe to mild Pain Nausea vomiting Accompanied swelling of the scrotum
Possible causes	Testicular trauma Testicular torsion Infection like epididymitis and orchitis Testicular tumors Inguinal hernia
Possible treatments	Testicular trauma: Pain medications, scrotal support, rest, occasionally surgery Testicular torsion: Emergency surgery for de-torsion Infection like epididymitis and orchitis: Pain medications, antibiotics, scrotal support, rest Testicular tumors: Surgery depending on the type of tumor Inguinal hernia: Surgery
Immediate action	Testicular pain requires immediate diagnosis with regards to its cause and in case of testicular torsion immediate de-torsion manually and surgically. Time is of the essence for such cases.
Prognosis	Testicular trauma: Good Testicular torsion: The quicker the surgery, the better the prognosis. Infections like epididymitis and orchitis: Very good Testicular tumors: Depends on the type and extent of the tumor Inguinal hernia: Very good

6 Testicular Infections: Pathogens can Affect the Testes

Depending on the location of an infection, medical literature distinguishes the following types of inflammation or infection in or around the male testis: an Epididymitis which affects the epididymis (see Figure 7, page 17), which is a rather small structure attached to the testes. To differentiate from this, an inflammation or infection that strikes the testicles themselves is called an Orchitis. Since the epididymis is in close proximity to the testes, infections often spread from here to the testicles resulting in a double infection called epididymo-orchitis.

Epididymitis

The epididymis is a tightly coiled tube on the rear side of each of your testis (see Figure 7, page 17). An infection of this "sperm storage" is often caused by bacterial invasions. In the tropical countries, filaria is its most common cause, closely followed by tuberculosis.

Most commonly, men between the ages of 20 to 39 suffer from this infection, although men of all ages are somewhat susceptible to it.

Symptoms

The symptoms of an acute epididymitis usually begin gradually and climax within 24 hours. The following list describes the common symptoms of this infection:

- Gradual onset of groin or scrotal pain. The pain level can range from mild to severe, and the intensity is often cyclical in nature, lasting from less than an hour to several days. Very often, one side of the groin or testis is more painful than the other side.
- Redness and warmth of the scrotum.

- Pain in the flank or abdomen.
- Swelling around the scrotum. The epididymis can swell to twice its size in a matter of 3-4 hours. It is worth mentioning that this swelling often varies from one patient to the other and can be accompanied by a hardening of the epididymis.
- Painful urination. Occasionally, blood may also be present in the urine.
- Urethral discharge at the tip of the penis. This symptom is much more common in men below 39 years of age with epididymitis.
- Fever with or without chills
- Nausea

In case of a chronic epididymitis, pain may be the only symptom.

Causes

Several possible factors are seen to cause epididymitis. Among them, bacteria is the most common cause of this infection, followed by viruses.

Bacterial causes:

Bacteria are prone to enter the epididymis in a retrograde direction from the urethra through the Vas Deferens and, lastly, into the epididymis. These bacteria are largely classified into two groups, sexually transmitted organisms, and coliforms.

Coliforms are the bacteria found in the gut or intestines. Some examples would be the Escherichia coli (E.coli) bacteria, staphylococci, and streptococci. These same organisms cause frequent bladder or urinary infections too. Not surprisingly, men indulging in anal intercourse are more susceptible to contracting such bacterial infections, which includes bladder infections and epididymitis.

Men younger than 39 years of age are more likely to catch infections due to sexually transmitted organisms, whereas men above this age have an increased risk of epididymitis caused by coliforms. Among the sexually transmitted organisms, the Chlamydia trachomatis causing the Chlamydia infections is responsible for 50-60% of the epididymitis cases. The bacteria causing gonorrhea including Neisseria gonorrhea result in the rest of them.

Viral causes:

Viral epididymitis is usually seen in the pediatric age group. Its most common cause is a mumps infection that travels down to the testes.

Chemical epididymitis:

This rare form of epididymitis is a result of backward or retrograde flow of urine from the urethra to the epididymis. Such an occurrence is likely to arise when one indulges in exercise or sexual intercourse on an overfull bladder.

Medications:

Amiodarone, a medication frequently used for heart conditions can possibly cause inflammation of the epididymis as an undesired side effect.

Diagnosis

The diagnosis of epididymitis including its causative organisms is important, as an incorrect diagnosis will only worsen the condition in affected individuals. Hence, a healthcare professional will take a detailed history and conduct a thorough physical exam if he/she suspects epididymitis. One of the characteristics of epididymitis is that, in addition to the symptoms described above, the cremasteric reflex (elevation of the testicle in response to stroking the upper inner thigh) is not changed.

Besides the physical exam, the following laboratory tests and imaging techniques aid in the diagnosis of this condition:

- Urine analysis and urine culture for urinary infections and STDs.

- Urethral culture: a swab may be inserted one and a half inches inside the urethra and sent for testing.
- A complete blood count to look for the white blood cell count. A high white blood cell count indicates the presence of an infection.
- Gram staining of the urethral exudates to detect the causative organisms.
- Ultrasound of the groin and pelvis to rule out testicular torsion, hydrocele, hernias, and abscesses.

It is essential to diagnose epididymitis correctly because in cases of sexually transmitted infections, the sexual partner needs to be notified about precautionary measures, testing, and medications too. The sexual partners are advised to undergo tests for STDs, use barrier contraceptives during sexual intercourse, and refrain from oral sex. Sometimes, a course of antibiotics as a preventive measure is prescribed for the sexual partner too.

Treatment

Conventional therapy

The treatment for epididymitis depends on its causative organisms. In most cases, the healthcare professional prescribes antibiotics for a span of 10 days or more. The choice of antibiotics and the route of administration, whether oral or intravenous, would depend on the severity of the infection.

Here's a list of antibiotics commonly used in the treatment of epididymitis infections:

Ceftriaxone:

A single dose of this antibiotic is given intravenously or intramuscularly in men below 39 years of age. Usually, ceftriaxone is accompanied by one dose of azithromycin, another antibiotic. Men above 39 years of age are often prescribed ciprofloxacin pills and Sulfamethoxazole and trimethoprim pills twice a day for 10-14 days.

Doxycycline:

Doxycycline is given orally, in addition to the ceftriaxone injection. The Centers for Disease Control and Prevention (CDC) guidelines suggest a ceftriaxone 250 mg single dose intramuscularly coupled with doxycycline 100 mg twice orally for 10 days.

Levofloxacin:

The CDC guidelines recommend levofloxacin 500 mg orally once a day for a span of 10 days to treat epididymitis in men who do not have a STD infection.

Apart from the antibiotics, the pain is treated with over-the-counter nonsteroidal anti-inflammatory drugs or NSAIDs like ibuprofen, naproxen, or acetaminophen.

Treatment guidelines and mode of treatment is likely to change frequently depending on many factors. Hence, do not try to self-treat your epididymitis but trust the discretion of your physician.

Alternative therapies

Ayurvedic and homeopathic treatments for epididymitis would be the same as mentioned under Alternative Therapy for testicular pain (see page 39).

Prognosis

The prognosis of epididymitis is excellent if detected and treated appropriately. The pain is likely to reduce in 2-3 days once the treatment with antibiotics begins; but the swelling is likely to take several days to go away.

The longer one delays the treatment of epididymitis, the chances of complications such as sterility, abscess, sepsis, or spread of the infection to the bloodstream, and epididymo-orchitis or spread of infection to the testes, increase further.

Orchitis

Orchitis is the infection of one or both of the testes in men. It usually results from the spread of bacteria through the blood to the testicles from other locations in the body. The most common example of this is the spread of an epididymitis infection to the testes known as an epididymo-orchitis infection. Another common cause of orchitis is the mumps virus in children which spreads from the parotid glands to the testicles. Since the testes are so closely connected to the epididymis, testicular infection or orchitis is very similar to epididymitis in its symptoms, causes, diagnosis, and treatment patterns.

Symptoms

The following symptoms are seen in orchitis:

- Rapid onset of pain in one or both the testes that is likely to spread to the groin.
- The affected testes are tender to touch, swollen, and may appear red or purple.
- A feeling of discomfort or heaviness may be present around the affected testis.
- Occasionally, blood in semen (hematospermia) may be present depending on the extent of the infection. Now and then, blood may be present in the urine too.
- High fever with nausea and vomiting maybe a sign of an underlying orchitis.
- Painful urination, pain in the groin from straining to pass motion, pain during sexual intercourse, and weakness are some accessory symptoms of orchitis.
- Pain or burning before or after passing urine, and penile discharge is also present in some men.

Epididymo-orchitis also appears with similar symptoms.

The symptoms of orchitis are similar to those of testicular torsion (page 52), so one may confuse both of them quite easily.

Causes

The causes of orchitis are the same as those mentioned under epididymitis (see page 45).

Diagnosis

Orchitis is diagnosed with the same techniques and tests as the epididymitis infections (see page 46).

Treatment

The treatment of orchitis or epididymo-orchitis is similar to epididymitis treatment programs, since the causative factors of both of these infections are the same (see page 47).

Additionally, using snug-fitting underwear or good scrotal supporters or athletic jock straps is likely to reduce the pain and discomfort from orchitis. Scrotal support is helpful as it reduces friction and movement of the scrotum by keeping it fixed in one position.

Prognosis

The outlook of orchitis is good if the infection is treated with antibiotics and appropriate medications promptly. On the contrary, a delay in treatment may result in the shrinking and decrease of function of the affected testis. Untreated orchitis may also lead to possible infertility and overall loss of the affected testis.

Quick summary of testicular infection

Condition	Testicular Infection
Main symptoms	Pain in the groin, flanks, and scrotum Nausea and vomiting Fever with chills Discoloration of the affected testicle
Possible causes	Bacterial: Chlamydia trachomatis, Neisseria gonorrhea, E. Coli, staphylococci, streptococci, etc. Viral: mumps virus Chemical: sexual intercourse or exercise with an overfull bladder. Drugs: Amiodarone
Possible treatments	Antibiotics, e.g. Ceftriaxone, Azithromycin, Doxycycline, Levofloxacin OTC pain medications, e.g. Naproxen, Ibuprofen, Acetaminophen Ice packs, rest, scrotal support
Immediate action	Diagnostic tests and antibiotic therapy
Prognosis	Very good

7 Testicular Torsion: What is it and why does it call for Immediate Action?

Testicular torsion is a surgical emergency and requires prompt medical intervention. The testes are suspended in the scrotal pouch by the spermatic cord on the top. They are further moored in place by a layer of skin that surrounds them from all sides, the tunica vaginalis. The cord contains the artery and vein that form the major blood supply of the testicle it holds in place. Just like any other organ or region in your body, your testes cannot survive without blood, which provides them with essential oxygen.

Testicular torsion occurs when the spermatic cord and the tunica vaginalis twist around themselves. As a result, the blood supply to the affected testes gets cut off, eventually exposing the testicles to harm due to lack of blood and oxygen.

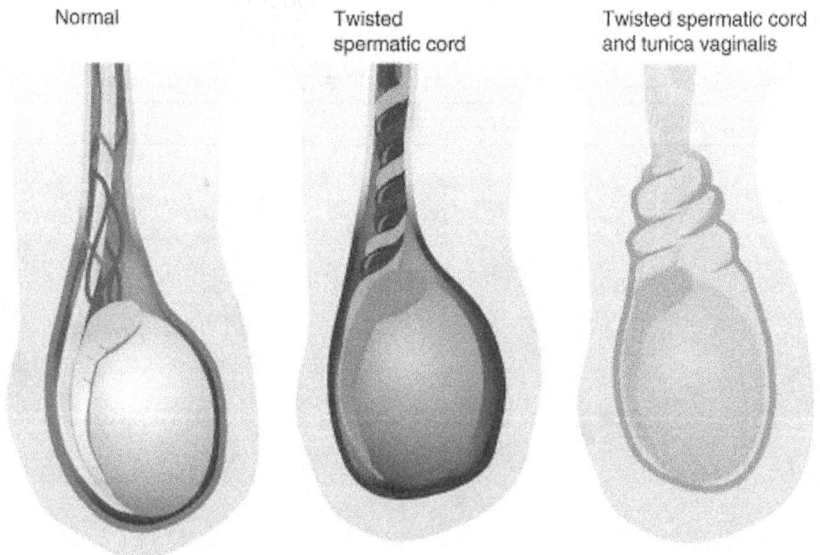

Figure 13: Testicular Torsion

(Source: OpenI)

Testicular torsion is an extremely painful condition and the leading cause of testicular loss in adolescent males. This condition affects as many as 1 in 4000 males below 25 years of age every year [7]. Most cases of testicular torsion occur in males below 30 years of age, with an increased frequency in adolescents between the ages of 12-18 [8].

Severe and sudden pain in the groin is usually the first and only indication of testicular torsion. Most healthcare professionals begin treatment for this condition based on symptoms and suspicion alone, as there isn't always enough time to wait for the results of the diagnostic tests, because testicular torsion requires immediate surgical correction to salvage the affected testes by resuming its blood supply.

Causes

The most common cause of testicular torsion is an anatomical malformation known as the bell-clapper deformity. In this condition, the tunica vaginalis covering the testis attaches to the spermatic cord at a point higher than normal. As a result, the testis rotates freely in the scrotum. This gives the spermatic cord more scope to twist around itself, resulting in a cut-off of the testicular blood supply. Usually, the bell-clapper deformity is present on both the sides, which makes both testes susceptible to torsion. To put it simply, imagine a puppet suspended on strings. Just as a puppet is susceptible to rotating along its strings, so are the ill-attached testicles susceptible to rotation along the spermatic cords.

Testicular torsion can occur spontaneously or because of trauma, especially in the presence of the bell-clapper deformity.

Symptoms

Even though the most prominent symptom of testicular torsion is severe and sudden pain in the groin on the affected side, there is a complete set of signs and symptoms that help the healthcare professional diagnose this condition.

Here's a list of the most common symptoms that are likely to be present with testicular torsion:

- Excruciating and sudden one-sided testicular pain.
- Sudden swelling of the scrotal pouch on the affected side.
- The affected testicle is often elevated higher than the adjoining testicle.
- The pain may even radiate up to the abdomen and pelvis.
- Testicular torsion often causes nausea and vomiting, too.
- Fever may be present with the rest of the symptoms of testicular torsion.

Diagnosis

Testicular torsion is diagnosed with a careful physical examination of the groin. Typically, a painful scrotum with a unilateral testicular swelling and elevation points to a testicular torsion diagnosis.

The healthcare professional may also perform a urine analysis and complete blood count.

Imaging with a Doppler ultrasound of the testes or a nuclear scan using a radioactive dye of the testes may also be carried out to assess the degree of blood loss to the affected testes.

All said and done, remember that testicular torsion requires immediate surgery, so not all cases are likely to undergo investigation. In most cases, the healthcare professional looks at the signs and symptoms, and diagnoses testicular torsion on a degree of suspicion alone.

Treatment

Conventional treatment

The treatment for testicular torsion is immediate surgery to bring about de-torsion of the affected testis and restart its blood flow. The surgeon may at first try to correct the twisted spermatic cord manually, before going in for surgery. The first and foremost objective of surgery for testicular torsion is to salvage the affected testis. Once the surgeon is successful in bringing about the de-torsion of the testis and spermatic cord, the testicle is then sutured within the scrotum to avoid future twisting. This part of the surgery is known as orchiopexy. Unfortunately, this isn't always possible. In cases where the testis cannot be salvaged, it is removed entirely with a procedure known as orchiectomy.

Testicular torsion can be treated only with immediate surgery; there are no medications for this condition. As for the pain, patients are frequently given narcotics like morphine for symptomatic relief.

Alternate therapy

In a case of testicular torsion, the survival of the affected testicle is of utmost importance. And, the only way to do this is quick diagnosis and immediate surgery to de-torse the affected testicle. And so, it isn't prudent to try any medications or alternative therapies for this condition.

Prognosis

The prognosis of testicular torsion depends on the time elapsed from the onset of the symptoms to the successful de-torsion of the testis, manually or surgically. The chances of saving the testis reduce drastically with time. The quicker the spermatic cord is untwisted and testis de-torsed, the better the outlook and recovery for the testis.

Time elapsed between symptom onset to de-torsion	Rate of salvaging the testis
Within 6 hours	90-100%
After 12 hours	20-50%
After 24 hours	0-10%

Fertility is still maintained even after orchiopexy. Additionally, as long as one of the testes is unaffected, fertility remains unaffected to a great extent, even if the other testis is damaged or removed. If the de-torsion isn't carried out on time, testicular torsion is likely to result in complications such as loss of the affected testis, permanently damaged testis, infertility, and/or infection.

Quick summary of testicular torsion

Condition	Testicular Torsion
Main symptoms	Excruciating one-sided pain in the groin Affected testicle is slightly elevated Nausea and vomiting Fever
Possible causes	Bell-clapper deformity
Possible treatments	Emergency orchiopexy or orchiectomy surgery
Immediate action	Manual untwisting of the spermatic cord followed by emergency surgery
Prognosis	The quicker the surgery, the better the prognosis

8 Testicular Lumps and Swelling

A testicular lump is a swelling or a growth in one or both of the testes. One might intuitively think that such a lump is dangerous and most likely a malignant tumor (i.e. cancer), but in the majority of cases, this is not true. There are various causes for lumps within the scrotal bag or on the testes.

The following rule of the thumb can serve as a starting point, but it by no means replaces a thorough exam and diagnosis. Usually, testicular cancer lumps are painless. Hence, a painful lump on a testis is most likely something else. But, this isn't a certainty, as some men may experience pain with testicular tumors too. A majority of the testicular lumps are due to benign causes which may not even require treatment. Cancer Research UK estimates that less than 4 in every 100 testicular lumps are actually testicular cancer [9]. All said and done, it is always better to investigate a testicular lump carefully, just to make sure it isn't a serious medical condition.

Several possible factors may cause swelling or a lump on your testes, the most common being varicoceles, hydroceles, benign testicular tumors, and spermatoceles. In many cases these testicular lumps do not require treatment unless they cause pain, discomfort, and/or other damaging symptoms.

Testicular cyst/ Spermatocele

A spermatocele or spermatic cyst is an abnormal cyst in the epididymis. The epididymis is a compactly coiled tube connected to the testes responsible for transferring the sperm into the Vas Deferens (see Figure 7, page 17). Such cysts are noncancerous and are likely to cause no pain. A spermatocele is basically a sac that contains clear or milky fluid and sperm. Since these cysts tend to be painless; they may remain undetected until one examines the scrotum and testes for lumps. Spermatoceles typically appear after puberty and reach their maximum incidence in the group between 40 and 60 years of age.

Symptoms

Spermatoceles rarely cause any significant signs and symptoms. They often remain unproblematic and stable in size. However, large spermatoceles might result in the following symptoms:

- Pain or discomfort around the affected area
- A lump or fullness behind and above the affected testis
- Heaviness in the testicle that has the spermatocele

Causes

The cause behind the development of a spermatocele is not yet known properly. It's highly possible that they may result from a block in one of the many tubes of the epididymis. Then again, trauma and inflammation may also result in these cysts.

Diagnosis

A spermatocele is diagnosed with a through physical examination of the groin. In addition, your doctor may also perform a trans-illumination test to locate the spermatocele. This test is performed by shining a torch over the scrotum. The light helps diagnose if the mass is fluid-filled or solid. A fluid-filled mass increases the possibility of a spermatocele.

Finally, your healthcare professional may ask for an ultrasound of the groin. This imaging technique helps diagnose a spermatocele by ruling out any of the other pathologies that could cause a lump on the testis.

Treatment

Conventional Treatment

A spermatocele will not disappear by itself, but it may hardly require any treatment. Generally, spermatoceles don't cause any pain or symptoms, and so they can be left alone. But, if such a cyst turns large or painful, it will require treatment with pain medication and surgery.

- *Pain medication:* Over-the-counter pain medication like acetaminophen or ibuprofen is commonly used to relieve pain from a growing spermatocele.
- *Surgery:* A so-called Spermatocelectomy is performed using local or general anesthesia to remove a spermatocele. An incision is made over the scrotum and the spermatocele is separated from the epididymis. After surgery, a gauze-filled scrotal athletic supporter is used to protect and apply pressure over the incision. Possible complications of this surgery include reduced fertility from damage to the epididymis. Despite best surgical efforts, spermatoceles commonly return after surgery.
- *Aspiration and sclerotherapy:* This is a very infrequently used method in the treatment of spermatoceles. The fluid is removed from the cyst by aspiration with a special needle. The cyst is then injected with an irritating chemical that causes scarring of the sac and prevents the spermatocele from coming back. Since this method holds the risk of damaging the epididymis, it is used only in men past their reproductive years.

Alternate Therapy

Most spermatoceles do not require surgery. These types of cysts, although painless, can be treated with alternative therapy or natural remedies. More importantly, you don't want that cyst to grow any further, and that's where alternative therapy is likely to help. Most of these therapeutic methods effectively stall the growth of the spermatocele. In fact, they may even help you get rid of the cysts altogether.

Ayurveda and herbs

The following herbal cures are deemed effective in treating spermatoceles:

- Pumpkin seeds prevent and heal most cysts in the testes. Boil a handful of the pumpkin seeds in water and consume this infusion while still warm.
- Tomatoes contain lycopenes well known for their anti-oxidant properties. It's because of the lycopenes that tomatoes are linked with a lower risk of cyst formation.

Despite that fact that most herbs and natural remedies are harmless, consult your doctor before you take any herbs to make sure they are safe for you, especially if you have a serious or major underlying medical condition. Some herbs are known to interact with allopathic or conventional medications, or cause side effects.

Homeopathy

The first choice of treatment in homeopathy for spermatoceles is Apis mellifica 30. If this remedy fails to reduce the swelling, Graphites 6X is the next choice. Other remedies used to treat spermatoceles are Phytolacca and Sepia. Consult a homeopathic physician for the appropriate dosage and remedy for best results.

Prognosis

The outlook of a spermatocele is excellent in most cases, as it remains as a painless and symptomless lump. Even after surgical excision of such cysts, the outlook and recovery of the patients are very good. However, these cysts tend to recur even after surgery.

Varicocele

A varicocele is an enlarged vein anywhere within the scrotal pouches (see also Figure 3, page 12). They are very much like the varicose veins that we commonly see on the legs and feet. Veins are the blood vessels that transport the "used" blood, which has already delivered oxygen and nutrition to a specific region of the body and now is on the way back to the heart, to be pumped into the lungs and into a new circulation through the body. Since many veins go upwards in the body (when a person stands), they have "valves" that prevent the blood from flowing backwards in the pauses of the heart's pumping rhythm. When some of these valves no longer function properly, the backward flow increases the blood pressure in the affected vein locally, which in turn can lead to a widening of a vein in a certain region. If the vein tissue is somewhat flexible or weak, which is often hereditary, it allows the formation of the typical sacs full of dark (i.e. used) blood, which are often visible through the skin and are commonly called varix or varicose veins.

The enlargement of the veins in the scrotum develops gradually over time and is likely to affect the sperm production in the testes, subsequently affecting fertility. In young boys, a varicocele may even cause the testes to shrink or remain under-developed. Varicoceles are relatively easy to diagnose and most of them don't require treatment.

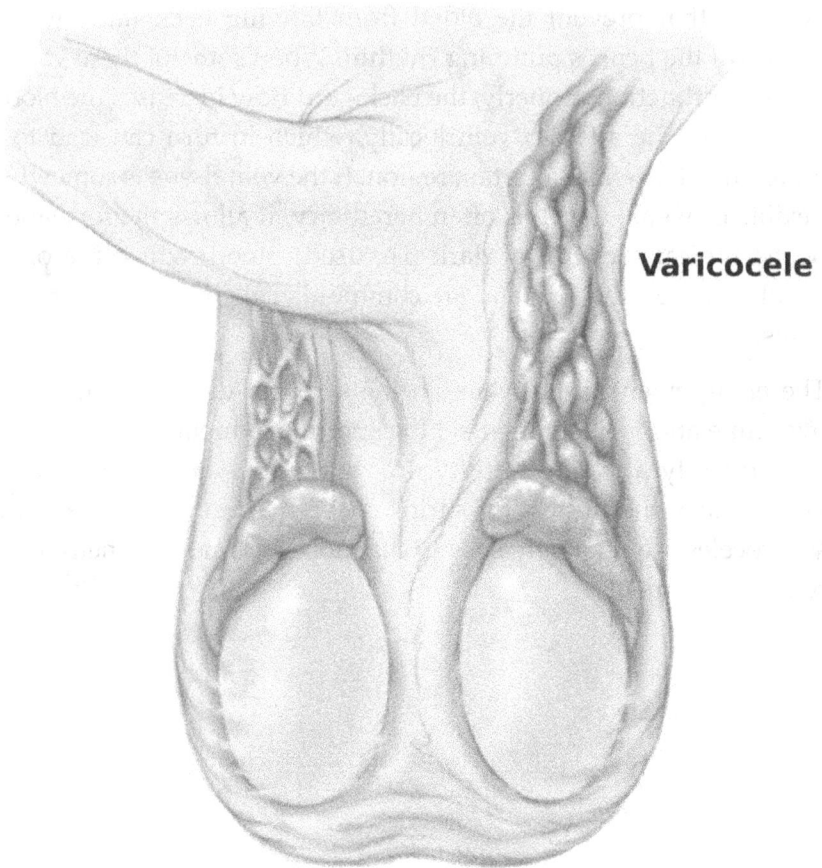

Varicocele

Figure 14: Schematic picture of a varicocele on the left side (from patient perspective)

(Source: OpenI)

Symptoms

Varicoceles usually don't produce any uneasy symptoms. However, as they increase in size, they may begin to cause pain and discomfort. The following symptoms are typical for varicoceles:

- A swelling which feels like a bag of worms around the affected testicle
- Most of the varicoceles are on the left side, probably due to the position of the left testicle. This "nut" is generally lower

than the right, which makes the left spermatic vein longer and more susceptible to dysfunctional valves because it has to work harder against gravity to take the blood from the left testicle to the heart, as compared to the right spermatic vein. Also, the left renal vein is compressed near the left kidney; this results in a pressure build-up in the left internal spermatic vein as it moves the blood from the left testicle to the heart through the left renal vein. This is known as the "nutcracker effect"

- Pain that varies from a sharp to dull discomfort.
- Pain increases throughout the day.
- Pain increases on standing or from physical exertion for longer periods. Pain decreases when lying on the back.
- Younger men may have impaired sperm production and testicular development from a varicocele.

A varicocele in one testicle is likely to affect sperm production in both the testes.

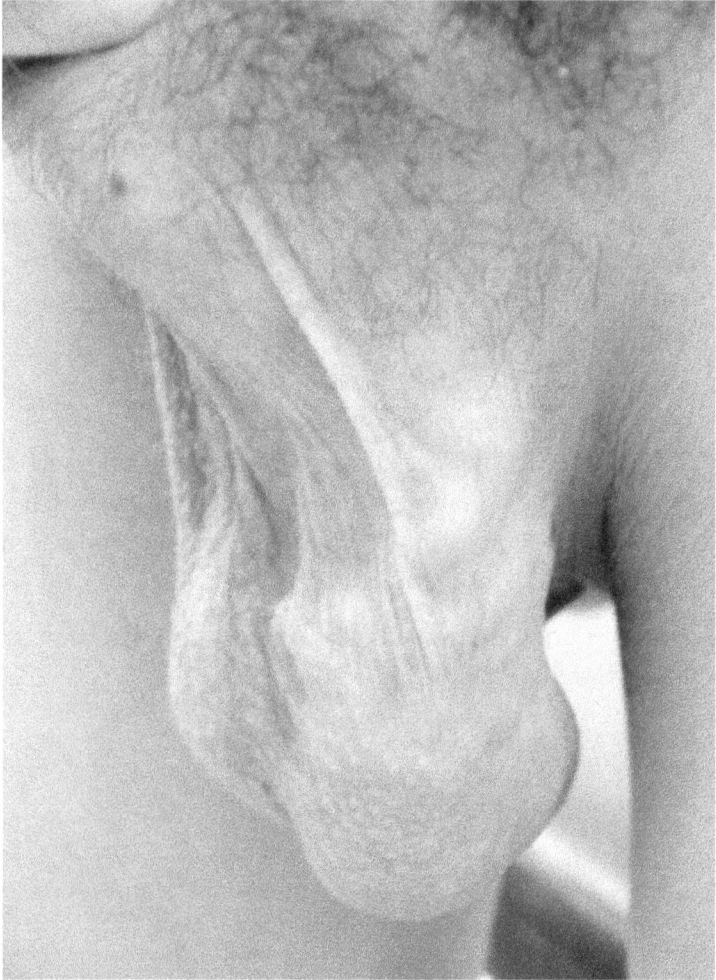

**Figure 15: Picture of a big varicocele which is clearly visible through
the scrotal skin**

(Source: OpenI)

Causes

The causative factors of varicoceles aren't known. Some experts believe that a local malfunctioning of the valves within the spermatic veins that travel through the spermatic cord is likely to result in this condition. Dysfunctional valves may result in an abnormal blood flow in these veins which in turn leads to a widening of the veins, which is causative for this condition.

Diagnosis

A physical examination of the scrotum is generally enough to diagnose a varicocele. On examination, the varicocele appears like a non-tender mass above the testis which feels like a bag of worms. In the case of smaller varicoceles or inconclusive physical examinations, the healthcare professional may ask for a scrotal ultrasound to diagnose this condition.

Treatment

Conventional Treatment

Most varicoceles may not require any treatment. But, when a varicocele causes testicular atrophy, pain, or infertility, the healthcare professional may recommend surgery to seal off the affected vein. As a result, the blood is redirected through the adjoining normal veins. Surgical options for varicocele include open surgery, laparoscopic surgery, and percutaneous embolization.

Alternate Therapy

Varicoceles are generally left alone by conventional medicine, unless they are capable of irreparable harm to the affected testicle. In distinction, alternative therapy often helps reduce the pain and other symptoms from a varicocele, in addition to gradually decreasing its size.

Ayurveda and herbs

- The herb Ashwashila is well known as a treatment for varicoceles.
- Mukkuti leaves are also believed to treat this condition. Steep 20 mukkuti leaves in around 300 ml of boiling hot water for 40 minutes. Strain the infusion and drink it twice a day for a month for positive results.

- 1 teaspoon of psyllium seed husk fiber added to your food daily is supposed to help with a varicocele.
- Butcher's broom and Horse chestnut effectively improve the tone and functioning of the testicular veins.

You can easily find these herbs in an ayurvedic store or from an herbalist. Some of them are also available on the internet. However, make sure you buy only authentic and quality herbs for better results. Consult your doctor before taking these herbs, especially if you have an underlying medical illness.

Homeopathy

Pale and anemic men with varicocele pain which gets worse with pressure and is better with application of cold or ice packs are likely to improve with Ferrum phos 6C. Whereas, testicular pain from a varicocele which feels better with cold application but worse with heat or lying on the affected side may benefit from a few doses of Pulsatilla 6C. Another remedy for Varicocele is Hamamelis 6C. This remedy is recommended for men with severe pain which radiates to the abdomen. Hamamelis is also a good remedy for men with both varicocele and piles or hemorrhoids. Another homeopathic remedy that helps treat varicoceles is Tabaccum, both as globules and as a poultice for the scrotum. Flabby genital organs with reduced sexual desire and erections are the symptoms that indicate this one.

Prognosis

The prognosis of an untreated varicocele isn't very good, since it is likely to result in decreased sperm production in one or both the testes. In young boys, a varicocele may even hinder the growth and development of the testes, sometimes even resulting in shrinkage. Varicoceles also tend to keep the temperature in the scrotum too high, which isn't optimal for sperm development. Thus, they are likely to result in subsequent infertility.

Benign testicular tumors

Tumors are lumps or masses of different sizes that can come up anywhere in the body, even in the testicles. They are broadly categorized as cancerous or malignant on the one hand, and noncancerous or benign on the other hand. Most malignant tumors are painless, whereas most benign tumors are painful. However, that does not mean that a painful tumor isn't cancer. Since there are very often exceptions to the rules, some cancerous or malignant tumors cause pain as well. The malignant tumors usually have an ill-defined margin and are attached or stuck to the surrounding organs. So, if you hold a malignant tumor between two fingers during a palpation, it may not move easily, or it may not move at all. On the other hand, benign tumors are usually encapsulated within a well-defined margin, and also, they are not attached to any adjacent tissue or organ. So during a physical examination, they may move more freely if held between two fingers.

The majority of tumors of the testes are benign or non-cancerous in nature. Benign testicular tumors are of two types: leydig cell tumors, and sertoli cell tumors.

The leydig cell tumors arise from the interstitial cells of leydig interspersed within the connective tissue inside the testes (see Figure 6, page 16). These tumors often occur before puberty. Since the leydig cells are responsible for secreting testosterone, such a tumor causes excess production of this hormone. In line with the higher testosterone, increased muscular development and sexual precocity are common attributes among boys with these tumors.

The sertoli cell tumors arise from the sertoli cells in the lining of the seminiferous tubules (see Figure 6, page 16). These are usually post-puberty tumors and are likely to cause an increase in female hormones. Hence, symptoms like gynaecomastia (see Figure 16 below) or increased breast size, loss of libido, and aspermia (meaning no sperm production) are seen with these tumors.

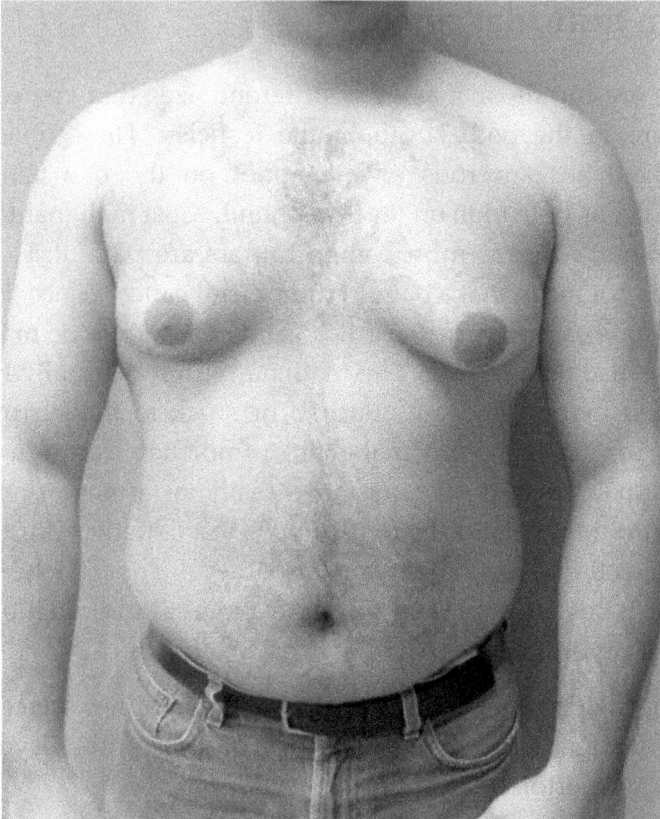

Figure 16: Adult male with severe gynaecomastia
(Source: By Dr. Mordcai Blau, CC BY-SA 3.0)

The diagnosis of benign testicular tumors is done with extensive imaging using scrotal ultrasonography and serum markers. Generally, surgery for such tumors is performed by specialized urologists and involves the removal of the tumor or the whole testicle. Recent advances in urology are now enabling surgeons to perform organ-sparing surgery on the affected testis, so that only the benign tumor mass is excised and not the entire testis [10].

Quick summary of testicular lumps and swellings

Condition	Testicular lumps and swellings
Main symptoms	A lump or mass on the testicle
Possible causes	Spermatocele, varicocele, benign testicular tumors, testicular cancer
Possible treatments	Surgical excision of the lump
Immediate action	Surgery if the lump is cancerous, painful, or affects fertility
Prognosis	Spermatocele: Excellent
	Varicocele: Medium to Good
	Benign testicular tumors: Good

9 Testicular Cancer

Cancer in all of its different forms is a widespread disease and a dominant topic in the media. The majority of people either have a friend or relative who is affected by cancer, or they even struggle with this threatening disease themselves, or did so in the past. In the light of the fact that cancer is such a big topic in our modern lives, when speaking with people, I am very often surprised about how little is known about the fundamental mechanism of this disease. Therefore, the following section is meant to lay the groundworks for understanding cancer in general, before taking a closer look at the specifics of testicular cancer.

What is Cancer in general?

A human body is made up of trillions of cells, each with a specific function, that synergistically cooperate to bring about a real miracle: this is that we are alive. This enormously complex system renews itself in every moment of its existence by creating new cells through cell division, which in time, mature and fulfil their specific roles. Over time, these cells "grow old" and finally die. This final step is initiated by a program of self-termination called **apoptosis** [11] (programmed cell death). During their lifespan, our cells are confronted with a variety of harmful, influential factors that they can compensate to a certain degree. Examples of such influences are poisonous substances, microorganisms (bacteria, viruses), extreme temperatures, electricity, or different forms of radiation such as light, radioactivity, or microwaves, to name just a few. In case one or several of these influences gets too strong, the genes (DNA) of a given cell may be altered in a way that renders it useless but also possibly harmful to the overall organism. Such a change whether it be insignificant, beneficial, or harmful is labelled a *mutation*. Mutations happen often, and normally, the human body is capable of correcting most of these changes. A single alteration is unlikely to cause cancer, but the accumulation of several harmful mutations can cause a cell to become cancerous. Some of the mutated cells are still able to execute the apoptosis program, while others start to grow and divide uncontrolled. It is then up to our immune system to detect these "evil mutants" and kill them. The specific cells of our immune system that mainly carry out these "executions" are T-lymphocytes, which recognize and mark proteins or cells to be killed, and macrophages [12] (Greek: big eaters) that tear the marked "enemies" apart and literally eat them. Macrophages are also capable of producing toxic chemicals, such as nitric oxide, which can kill surrounding cells. It is estimated that every day of our life, millions of our body cells mutate and are subsequently either corrected or "eaten" by this type of white blood cell in a process called phagocytosis.

As long as our immune system is strong enough to kill the cancer-to-be mutant cells, we stay healthy. There are two factors that can endanger this dominance of our body's defense system:

- the harmful influences get too strong, and/or
- our immune system is, due to stress or an unhealthy lifestyle, too weak to kill all ill-mutated cells.

One or both factors may only be given in a certain region of our body and only within a limited timeframe. But this may suffice for ill-mutated cells to grow at high speed and to build structures which make them "invisible" to our immune system. They do so by building an immunosuppressive environment through producing "T-lymphocyte regulators" with which they deactivate the T-lymphocytes. This way, the T-lymphocytes do not recognize the cancer cells and cannot mark them as "enemies to be eaten". As a consequence they can go on growing, being fed by the blood stream, and form cancerous tumors. Their dangerous characteristic is that they grow at high speed and penetrate their environment, thereby causing damage to vital structures of our bodies. They might even send cancerous cells to other parts of our body and thus initiate the growth of further cancerous tumors, a process called metastasis.

Due to the gradual slowdown of cell division with increasing age, cancer usually grows slower in older people as compared to younger ones.

There are two fundamental strategies to treat cancer: one is to remove or kill the cancerous tissue by means of surgery, chemotherapy, or radiation, and the other is to strengthen our immune system so that it can destroy the cancer, or at least slow down or stop its further growth.

The specifics of testicular cancer

You have already learned in the previous chapters that the testes or the male gonads are located behind the penis in sac-like pouches or scrotal bags, and that they produce sperm and androgens or male hormones throughout a man's lifetime.

Testicular cancer is a malignant tumor of the testis, wherein certain cells within the testes become destructive and multiply uncontrollably.

Unlike most other cancerous diseases which mostly affect the geriatric age groups, testicular cancer is predominantly an ailment of young men. In fact, it is the most common type of malignant tumor affecting males between 20-39 years of age. As a relief for worried parents, this condition is rarely found in boys below 15 years of age. Fortunately, testicular cancer is curable in most cases and has a good prognosis in general. Yet, even the smallest of testicular lumps should be investigated thoroughly.

As mentioned in the previous chapter, not all testicular lumps are tumors, let alone malignant tumors. Although, testicular cancer occurs more frequently in young men than in other age groups, its prevalence isn't very high in the general population. In the United States alone, approximately 8,400 cases of testicular cancer are diagnosed every year. Testicular cancer accounts for only 1% of all cancers in American men and has resulted in 380 deaths in the US in 2014 [13]. In the UK, the official statistics count 2,207 new cases of testicular cancer in 2011. The crude incidence rate shows that there are 7 new testicular cancer cases for every 100,000 males in the UK [1]. In general, a man's risk of developing testicular cancer in his lifetime is between 1 in 200 and 1 in 263 [14]. Globally, testicular cancer accounted for 8300 deaths in 2013. Racially, testicular cancer incidences are 4-5 times higher in white males as compared to those in black males. Similarly, white men have a 3 times higher chance of testicular cancer as compared to Asian men. A recent study found an increase of the incidence of testicular cancer in white adults within the USA from 12.41 cases in 100,000 in 1992 to 13.22 in 2010. Astonishingly, but yet unexplained is a sharp rise of this condition in Hispanic whites in the US between 15 to 39 years of age from 7.18 to 11.34 within the same timeframe [15]. Overall, a man's lifetime risk of dying from testicular cancer is about 1 in 5000 [13].

The following charts show the development of the average statistical occurrence (incidence rate, IR) of testicular cancer, as well as the fraction of those who have died due to this disease (mortality rate, MR) for ten countries: chart A displays the IR for the time between 1958 and 2002; chart B depicts the MR in the period between 1955 and 2009. Chart C shows the annual changes in both incidence (left bar) and mortality rate (right bar) per country. Even though it is difficult to tell the different lines apart in the upper two charts, one can see the overall trend that the incidence rate increases in many countries; however, the mortality rate is low and decreases in the majority of the countries, most likely due to improved treatment [16].

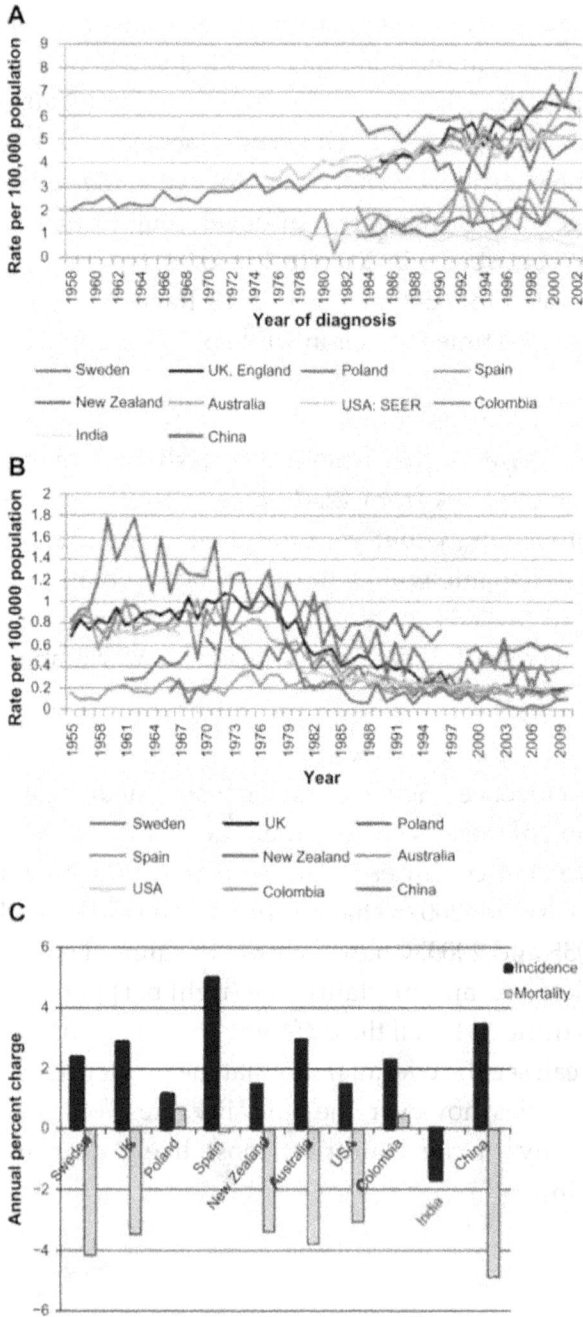

Figure 17: Testicular cancer incidence and mortality in 10 countries

Testicular cancer tumors are broadly classified as seminomas and non-seminomas according to the type of tumor cells they contain [17]. About 40% of the malignant testicular tumors are seminomas. These tumors are called "adenocarcinomas" that arise from the lining of the seminiferous tubules in the testes (see Figure 6, page 16). Adenocarcinomas are cancers that develop from glands or glandular tissues. Since the testicles are the male glands or gonads, tumors arising from the testes are often of the adenocarcinomic type. The seminomas are further classified as classic, anaplastic, and spermatocytic. The other varieties of malignant testicular tumors are the non-seminomas that arise from the primitive totipotent germ cells within the developing testes. These cells are purely embryonic in nature. The non-seminomas are further classified as choriocarcinomas, embryonal carcinomas, teratomas, and yolk sac tumors. Out of these, the teratomas account for 32% of the malignant testicular tumors. Some of the testicular tumors contain both seminoma as well as nonseminoma cells. Generally, teratomas affect younger men in the age group of 20-25, whereas seminomas affect men in the 30-35 years age group. All of this information may seem confusing to read. If it's all gone over your head, don't worry about it. What is important to remember are the different names by which these tumors are known.

Let's put all of these different tumors in a classification table for a better understanding of the different types of testicular cancers.

Classification and incidence of different forms of testicular cancer (TC)			
Seminomas (adenocarcinomas), 40-45% of all testicular cancers			
Subtypes:	Incidence in subgroup:	Age most affected:	Specifics:
Classical	85% - 95%	30-50	Slower growth than non-seminomas
Spermato-cytic	2-12%	Over 50, average around 65	Slower growth than classical seminomas
Anaplastic	5-10%	30-50	More aggressive
Non-seminomas, 55-60% of all testicular cancers			
Subtypes:	Incidence in subgroup:	Age most affected:	Specifics
Chorio-carcinomas	1-2%	n/a	Very Aggressive
Embryonal carcinomas	40% of all testicular cancers, but in pure form only in 3-4%.	25-35	Rapid growth and spreading outside of testicle
Teratomas	3% of adult testicular cancers and 38% of childhood testicular cancers	Childhood	Rarely spread to other organs
Yolk sac tumors	1-2%	most common form of TC in children (esp. in infants)	More serious in adults than in children.

Causes

The possible causes of testicular cancer are still largely unknown. But researchers have identified several factors that increase a man's risk of developing this disease. Some of the most important risk factors are listed and explained in the following.

Undescended testes or cryptorchidism

Males with an undescended testis have an increased risk of testicular cancer. Normally, the testes descend into their final position in the scrotum from the abdominal wall just before birth. Then again, 1-2 % of boys are born with an undescended testicle. This undescended testicle is expected to travel down sometime in the first year. Occasionally, the testicle may not descend down at all even after infancy. Such undescended testicles usually lie somewhere along the inguinal canal in the abdominal wall and have a higher risk of developing testicular cancer. Unfortunately, this risk does not go away even after surgical correction of the testicle's location. Furthermore, the increased risk of testicular cancer applies to both the testes alike [18].

Past history of testicular cancer

Men, who have had a malignant tumor in one of the testes, have an increased risk of developing testicular cancer tumors in the other unaffected testis, too.

Family history of testicular cancer

Testicular cancer is a familial disease. Its risk is higher among men who have first-degree relatives with testicular cancer. So, if your brother or father has had testicular cancer, you have an increased risk of developing such malignant tumors of the testes, too. In fact, the American Cancer Society recommends that men with a family history of testicular cancer should conduct a testicular self-exam every month to look for signs of a testicular tumor.

Congenital anomalies

Presence of anatomical abnormalities of the testes, penis, and kidneys are likely to increase a man's chances of developing testicular cancer. Additionally, inguinal hernias (see page 99) are also known to increase the risk of testicular cancer.

Chemicals, drugs, and supplements

Several substances from different origin (e.g. environmental, occupational, drug-based, or supplemental) have been found to raise the risk of developing testicular cancer (TC): For example, researchers have found that men who have detectable values of total polychlorinated organic compounds in their blood have a risk of 14.4% of getting TC as compared to 1% in those who do not have these substances in their bodies. So-called endocrine disruptors like certain pesticides, polychlorinated biphenyls (PCBs, used as coolants), or dibutyl phthalate (a chemical used to manufacture cosmetics, such as nail polish) are also suspected to increase the risk of TC [19]. A recent study showed that men who use muscle-building supplements (MBS) have a significantly elevated risk of developing testicular germ cell tumor (TGCT) as compared to those who do not consume MBS [20]. Similarly, the use of marijuana, even if consumed only once, has shown to have a 2-fold risk of developing TGCT as compared to people who have never used it [21].

Exposure to radiofrequency electromagnetic radiation

Radiofrequency electromagnetic radiation (RF-EMF) is emitted by many devices common in modern life, for example, mobile phones, cordless phones at home, wireless LAN devices such as notebooks and tablet computers, microwave ovens, radar stations for military and civil use, radio or television broadcasting stations, and many more. For a long time, it has been known that *in vitro* (which means in laboratory settings), RF-EMF of a certain magnitude causes mutations in human cells [22],[23]. Also *in vivo* (meaning in real-life settings), scientists have found that RF-EMF increases the risk of developing cancerous tumors [24], especially when the radiation lies above a certain threshold. When looking at the male reproductive system specifically, there is strong evidence from numerous studies that exposure to RF-EMF (specifically those emitted by mobile phones) is harmful in many respects [25], some of which being infertility and increased oxidative stress. The latter is a primary cause for cell mutations, which is the starting point for testicular cancer [26].

Symptoms

A testicular lump or swelling is the primary symptom of testicular cancer. It is also the first symptom noticed by the majority of patients. In most cases, the men themselves find such a lump on self-examination.

In general, patients often experience one or more of the following symptoms:

- A lump in one or both of the testes.
- In most cases, testicular cancer tumors are painless. Yet, it's essential to note that 1 in 4 of these tumors is painful. In these cases, patients describe their sensation as a sharp pain or a dull ache in the groin and lower abdomen.
- An abnormally enlarged testis.
- Heaviness in the groin or scrotum.
- Sudden filling up of the scrotum with fluid (also called hydrocele).
- Gynaecomastia or enlarged breasts in men due to increased secretion of the β-hCG hormone (see also Figure 16, page 68).
- Lower back pain is likely to arise when the tumor spreads to the lymph nodes at the back.
- Rarely, some patients present with chronic epididymo-orchitis (see also page 49) which fails to get better with medication.

Testicular cancer most commonly spreads to the lungs. However, it may also spread to other organs in the abdomen. Typical symptoms after metastasis or spread of testicular cancer to the lungs are:

- Breathlessness or dyspnea.
- Cough. Occasionally, the cough may be accompanied by blood or blood stained mucus.
- Lump in the neck from metastasis or spread of the malignant cells from the lungs to the cervical lymph nodes.
- Jaundice, ascites or fluid in the abdomen, hepatomegaly.

If you come across any lump or swelling on or around your testes, visit a healthcare professional to make sure it isn't testicular cancer. The medical fraternity looks upon any testicular lump in a young adult that may or may not be painful with suspicion, only to investigate it thoroughly. Although not all of these lumps are cancer, it's always better to be safe than sorry. That's why it is very important that you speak to your healthcare provider immediately if you suspect a testicular lump or swelling.

Staging of the testicular cancer tumors:

The testicular tumors are staged according to the TNM classification based on the guidelines published by the AJCC cancer-staging manual [27].

Stage I: Cancer cells localized to the affected testis

Stage II: Cancer cells metastasize or spread to the retroperitoneal and para-aortic lymph nodes located below the diaphragm. The diaphragm is a muscular sheet just below your lungs. It separates the chest cavity from the abdominal cavity.

Stage III: Cancer involving the testis that has spread beyond the retroperitoneal and para-aortic lymph nodes.

Diagnosis

Appropriate and prompt diagnosis of testicular cancer is of the utmost importance to halt the disease and its spread. Very often, its symptoms are mistaken with those of Hydrocele, Varicocele, and Epididymitis. In fact, a large number of testicular cancer cases go undiagnosed or they are misdiagnosed due to a lack of specific symptoms.

A thorough examination of the scrotal sacs and the testes reveals the presence of a lump or swelling in men with testicular cancer. These lumps are then investigated further with blood examinations and imaging to ascertain if they are malignant or something else:

- Scrotal ultrasound: The palpable lump on the testicle is investigated with an ultrasound of the scrotum to ascertain its type, nature, extent, and to look for poorly defined or circumscribed borders.

- CT scan: A computed tomography (CT) scan helps to ascertain the extent of the testicular cancer and metastasis to the other susceptible organs.

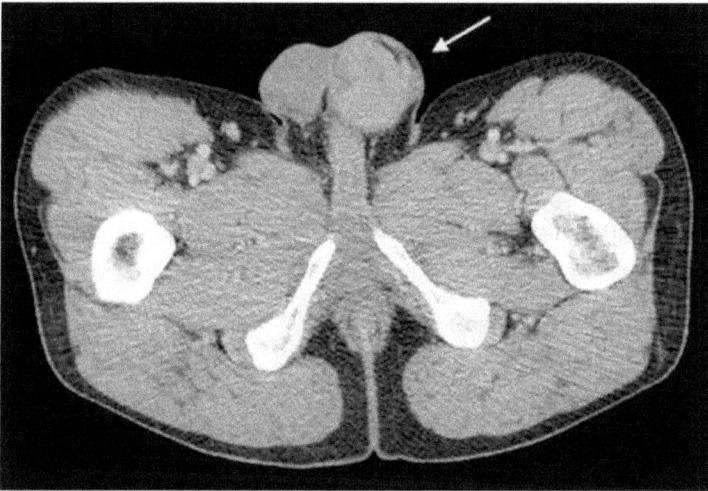

Figure 18: CT scan of a testicular tumor on the left side (see arrow)
(Source: OpenI)

- Tumor markers: These are blood tests that look for specific proteins which are likely to increase in the blood stream due to testicular cancer. Blood serum levels of alpha-feto protein, human chorionic gonadotropin or β-HCG, and LDH-1 are typically measured to diagnose testicular cancer. These levels are expected to be higher in patients with testicular cancer.

- Inguinal orchiectomy: This test replaces a biopsy in testicular cancer. It involves the removal of the entire testis with the attached Epididymis and spermatic cord. The testicular tissue is then studied to rule out testicular cancer. A mere biopsy that involves only partial removal of the testicle tissue is contra-indicated in testicular cancer. Mainly because a biopsy can lead to the cancer cells migrating to the back and abdominal wall through the lymphatic system, resulting in the spread of the cancer.

If any of these tests show the presence of testicular cancer, further tests are carried out to check the extent of the cancer and if it has spread to any of the other organs. Accordingly, the healthcare professional chalks out a treatment plan that best suits the patient.

Treatment

Standard treatment

The treatment of testicular cancer is made up of three pivotal aspects:

1. Surgery
2. Chemotherapy
3. Radiation therapy

Most patients with testicular cancer are cured of this disease with minimal long-term effects. The treatment success rate primarily depends on the stage of the cancer. The average survival rate of testicular cancers with treatment after 5 years is 95%. In fact, in stage I testicular cancers, the survival rate is as good as 100% [28]. This simply emphasizes why prompt action is essential when testicular cancer is suspected in a male.

The initial treatment of testicular cancer almost always involves surgical removal of the affected tissue. This surgery is usually followed by adjuvant therapy that includes chemotherapy or radiation, and careful surveillance of signs indicating a return of the testicular cancer. This combination is proving to be extremely successful in the treatment and recovery of patients with testicular cancer. Patients are also given the option of sperm banking before beginning with testicular cancer treatment, especially chemotherapy.

Surgery

Surgery is the first and most important step in testicular cancer treatment, mainly because it effectively gets rid of the cancerous cells. During surgery, the urologist removes the entire inner structure of a scrotal bag on the affected side (including testis, Epididymis, and the spermatic cord). This is ideally done through an incision below the belt-line on the abdomen. This procedure is known as *inguinal or radical orchiectomy*. The entire testicle and not just the tumor is removed because a partially eliminated testicle is likely to leave behind tumor-developing cells in the remaining part of the testes, increasing the risk of a recurrence. Since, one of the testes is enough to maintain fertility and the production of the male hormones, in almost all of the cases where testicular cancer is suspected, the entire affected testicle is removed for safety reasons. This surgery is sometimes followed by a retroperitoneal lymph node dissection (RPLND) to ascertain that no cancerous structures are left in the body if the testicular cancer has already spread. RPLND requires a higher level of expertise in the surgeon, and sperm banking itself can result in nerve damage that may cause the ejaculate to flow into the bladder instead of outside the urethra. As a result, most healthcare professionals prefer to use surveillance techniques instead of the RPLND surgery.

Adjuvant therapy

After surgery, the patient is given adjuvant treatment in the form of chemotherapy or radiation to prevent the spread of testicular cancer. The selection of such a therapy primarily depends on the type of tumor detected through histological studies of the testicle removed with surgery.

Radiation therapy

Radiation is mostly used as an adjuvant in stage 1 seminoma tumors alone, as it is ineffective against the nonseminoma tumors. It may result in side effects like fatigue, nausea, vomiting, diarrhea, and skin changes at the site where radiation is administered. Radiation also affects sperm production, although most patients regain their fertility after 1-2 years.

Chemotherapy

Nonseminoma: Chemotherapy is the standard treatment for nonseminoma tumors post-surgery. Three to four cycles of Bleomycin-Etoposide-Cisplatin is the preferred adjuvant therapy that works in halting the spread of nonseminoma tumors. Alternatively, four cycles of Etoposide-Cisplatin chemotherapy are also frequently used for this purpose.

Seminoma: Chemotherapy is gaining precedence over radiation in the treatment of seminoma testicular tumors too, since radiation seems to have more long-term side effects as compared to chemotherapy. Commonly, three doses of carboplatin are given three weeks apart as adjuvant therapy for seminoma tumors. Unfortunately, seminomas have a tendency to come back after many years. Hence, patients are advised to be vigilant and follow proper surveillance techniques even after five years have passed the first incidence of a seminoma testicular tumor.

Chemotherapy may cause several side effects like fever with chills, vomiting, nausea, diarrhea, fatigue, hair loss, skin rashes, oral ulcers, shortness of breath, and dizziness. Occasionally, it may also cause hearing impairment, numbness, and loss of reflexes. The chemotherapy drugs are moreover likely to affect sperm production and affect fertility. In most cases, the reduction in sperm count is permanent; nevertheless, many men have been known to regain their fertility after a few years.

Surveillance

The aim of surveillance in patients of testicular cancer post-surgery is to detect a relapse or metastasis as early as possible. Since, time is of the essence when it comes to treating and curing testicular cancer, surveillance is an important aspect of its treatment today.

For both seminomas and non-seminomas, surveillance regimens include physical examination, blood tests for tumor markers, CT scans of the abdomen and sometimes chest, and X-rays of the chest. The number of tests and their frequency is likely to vary depending on the type of testicular tumor. For instance, seminomas rarely show an increase in the tumor markers; hence, blood tests may not help much with their surveillance. The CT scan can help detect a relapse or spread of the tumors to the chest and abdomen, whereas the X-ray is quite successful in detecting a pulmonary metastasis by itself. In addition, a PET scan (Positron emission tomography) can be used to spot cancerous tissues and cells that may not always be found with computed tomography (CT) or magnetic resonance imaging (MRI). A PET scan reveals how the body is functioning and uncovers areas of abnormal metabolic activity.

Most cases of testicular cancer undergo surveillance for 5 years. Certain high-risk groups may even require surveillance for a longer period.

Alternate therapy

Testicular cancer is a curable disease, and in no way should its treatment be delayed. The best solution is the removal of the affected testicle. This strategy stops the growth of the tumor and its spread by literally nicking the disease in its bud.

Alternative therapy is more likely to help with providing relief from the symptoms of testicular cancer and in reducing the risk of its recurrence. All said and done, alternative therapy should not be looked at as a replacement for surgery. Before you begin taking any herbal preparations, speak to your doctor in case you are on other medications like chemotherapy, or you are currently being treated with radiation. Herbs are almost always harmless, yet they are medicines too and can increase or decrease the efficacy of some conventional medicines.

Most testicular tumors are asymptomatic in the initial stage, which means they silently grow inside your body without any overt signs or symptoms. Alternative therapy is likely to be of much more help in these stages of testicular cancer in stopping further growth of the tumors and in hindering the spread of the disease. However, in the advanced stages of testicular cancer which has or hasn't spread to other organs, alternative therapy works as palliative therapy alone. It helps to ease discomfort and symptoms like pain, burning, etc.

Ayurveda and herbs

In a case control study, the Divyajyot Ayurvedic Research Foundation in India protocolled and evaluated the results of 770 patients suffering from different kinds of cancer on ayurvedic treatment from Jan 2004 to Dec 2004 [29].

Out of the 770, 504 were patients with primary cancer (cancer that affects a single organ and which hasn't spread or metastasized). 13% of these patients were disease free; 20.3% were markedly improved; 65.27% were improved; and 0.9% remained uncured at the end of this study.

Among the 226 patients with secondary cancer (cancer that has spread to other organs), 12.03% were disease free; 18.04% were markedly improved; 68.79% were improved; and 1.12% remained uncured by the end of this study.

These figures show that Ayurveda has the potential to be an important tool in the treatment of testicular cancer, if used judiciously. Ayurvedic herbs like Divya sila sindura, Divya tamra bhasma, Divya abraka bhasma, Divya giloy sat, and divya arogya vati are commonly used in the treatment of cancers [30].

Some ayurvedic physicians also suggest regular yoga sessions to relieve mental and physical stress and anxiety due to testicular cancer and its treatment. A note of caution, always consult a qualified ayurvedic practitioner or a herbologist to know the best course of action for your testicular cancer.

Homeopathy

Homeopathy is a safe and beneficial therapy for most chronic diseases, including cancer. Many patients report that homeopathic remedies have helped them to improve the symptoms of testicular cancer and slow-down its progress and spread. In cases of chronic and deep-seated conditions, homeopathy reduces the recurrence of the disease.

Testicular cancer with symptoms which are worse at night, and nocturnal emissions or ejaculate stained with blood can get better with mercurius. Burning pains with hardening and swelling of the testicle is often treated with Thuja occidentalis. Nonetheless, treating cancer with homeopathy prescriptions based on the patient's constitution show more promise than the specifics prescribed according to the symptoms. Constitutional remedies are prescribed based on a thorough case taking that considers the overall physical and mental health of the patient, in addition to his personality type and physical appearance. This method of prescription also considers the inherent tendency of the patient to contact certain diseases as well as any other underlying medical conditions. Visit a qualified homeopathic physician to know the most suitable homeopathic remedy for your constitution.

Naturopathy

This therapy involves an integrated approach which includes nutritional adjustments, exercise, deep tissue massage, counseling, acupuncture, and stress management. It is usually done in conjunction with conventional or western medicine. Naturopathy helps to create the healthiest and most suitable environment possible, internally and externally, for the rapid improvement of the patient with testicular cancer.

Nutritional Therapy

The nutritional demands of every person are likely to differ depending on various factors like body type, race, underlying medical conditions, food intolerances and allergies, as well as metabolic rate. Hence, the nutritional adjustments for testicular cancer may vary from patient to patient. As a general direction, most patients are asked to increase their intake of fruits, vegetables, legumes, whole grains, yoghurt, poultry, and fish. These changes may be clubbed with nutritional supplements of Vitamins E and C, eicosapentaenoic acid (EPA) which is an omega-3 fatty acid, selenium, and beta-carotene. Patients with cancer often have very low blood levels of Vitamin D3, since the immune system uses up this vitamin in its struggle against the cancer. There is scientific evidence that the administration of high doses of Vitamin D3 can enable the immune system to cope better with cancer. There are even case reports of cancer remission due to high doses of Vitamin D [31–34].

A nutritionist specialized in cancer diets should be able to help you with your nutritional requirements.

Other alternative therapies

- Intense nutraceutical IV therapy, containing, for example, multiple vitamins, herbs, amino acids, minerals, chlorophyll, and hydrogen peroxide. These ingredients work together to re-enable the body of the patient to destroy the cancerous cells and provide nourishment to the healthy cells in the testicles and elsewhere.
- High dosage Vitamin C infusions have shown to selectively kill cancer cells [35, 36]. Linus Pauling, a Nobel laureate, was the first to propose this therapy in a 1976 study he conducted along with Ewan Cameron.

- Pyrroloquinoline Quinone (PQQ) is a substance that has the ability to induce apoptosis (programmed cell death, see also page 70) in cancer cells [37]. In other words, it leads cancer cells to "commit suicide," which is highly welcome. PQQ is available as prescription-free supplement, but it is recommended to consult your physician concerning dosage and possible cross effects with other medication or supplements.

- Hyperbaric Oxygen therapy (HBOT) is breathing 100% oxygen while under increased atmospheric pressure. As a result, the amount of oxygen in the blood increases, thereby also raising the pH level of the blood and consequently in all body tissues. This more basic (alkaline) and oxygen-rich environment is less conducive for the survival of the cancer cells. The fundamental principle of HBOT in cancer treatment goes back to Otto Warburg (Nobel laureate) who showed that oxygen is a natural enemy of cancer. Indeed, cancer cells thrive in oxygen-depleted environments with a low (i.e. acidic) pH (so-called hypoxic pockets). This environment seems to protect the cancer cells from the outside world, leaving them alone to burn glucose and flourish. Weakening or even taking away this protective environment by introducing more oxygen into the blood has the potential to stop the spread of the cancer through metastasis and even to reduce existing cancerous lumps [38].

- Mag heat ray therapy. This therapy works on the principle that the cancer cells may not survive at a temperature above 107 degrees Fahrenheit.

Speak to specialized healthcare providers about these therapies to learn if they are suitable for you, and be aware that not all of these have been comprehensively researched and verified for all of their beneficial effects and side effects. Hence, if you consider going for any of them, research them thoroughly and get at least a second opinion from an authentic and qualified practitioner.

Prognosis

The prognosis of most testicular cancers is promising. Improved surveillance and surgical techniques have only led to better prospects for testicular cancer patients. Regardless of the stage of the testicular tumor, a significantly improved and sustained response is seen in 90% of testicular cancer patients. In 2016, Cancer Research UK reported more than 96% of the 2300 men diagnosed with testicular cancer as cured. These better prognostic results are being attributed to superior surgical and surveillance techniques, and the chemotherapy drug, cistaplatin.

Fertility

Removal of one of the testes is not likely to affect male fertility, as long as the other testis is unaffected and healthy enough to produce sperm and testosterone normally. Even so, patients who wish to have children and are expected to have impaired fertility from removal of both testes, chemotherapy, or radiation, are frequently given the option of sperm banking. Sperm banking still gives the male the option of conceiving a child through IVF techniques. Only the removal of a single testis does not usually affect the man's sexual performance and sperm production. Such men are perfectly capable of conceiving children naturally, despite the removal of a single testicle.

Quick summary of testicular cancer

Condition	Testicular cancer
Main symptoms	Testicular lump, usually painless Heaviness in the groin
Possible causes	Cryptorchidism, familial tendency, anatomical abnormalities of the testis
Possible treatments	Surgery followed by radiation or chemotherapy

Immediate action	Diagnosis and surgical removal of the entire testicle
Prognosis	Very good to moderate, depending on stage

Preventive measures against testicular cancer are described in a separate section which starts on page 109.

Should you be generally worried or on the lookout for testicular cancer?

It's important for women to examine their breasts regularly for breast cancer lumps. We all know that, because breast cancer has received extensive publicity in the past and so have the breast exams. But, it's equally important for men to conduct a testicular self-exam. Not many men are aware of this fact, and so a considerable number of men realize they have testicular cancer rather late, sometimes even too late. Yet, the incidence of testicular cancer isn't as high as that of breast cancer, and not all testicular lumps are cancer.

It is no doubt better to be on the safe side: every male between 20-40 years of age should be on the lookout for testicular cancer. Usually, there isn't any need to panic over a small lump that may turn out to be something entirely harmless. Yet, it wouldn't hurt to be alert and pick up such lumps at the outset. Remember that testicular cancer is predominantly a medical condition of the young and not the elderly.

The American Urological Association recommends that young men should self-examine their scrotum and testes for lumps on a monthly basis. Additionally, the American Cancer Society also suggests a monthly testicular self-examination in men who have a high risk of testicular cancer. Mainly, they suggest that men with family members with testicular cancer, or a history of this condition in themselves, should be extra vigilant.

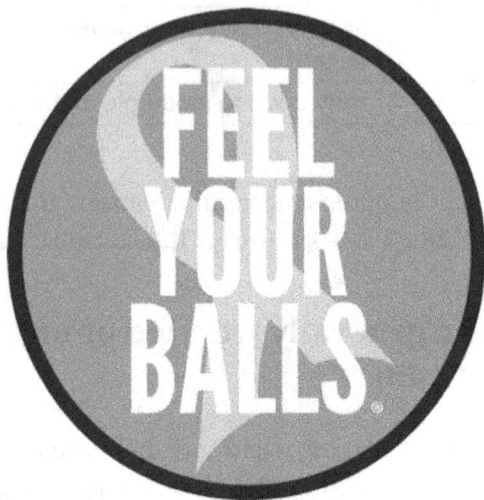

If a self-exam of your testicles reveals a testicular lump or an abnormal finding, consult a healthcare professional before you panic or form unwanted misconceptions in your mind. Less than 4 in 100 testicular lumps or swellings are actually malignant, but it never hurts to err on the side of caution.

Watching out for testicular lumps is essentially important, as early detection of any testicular pathology, especially malignant lumps, holds a better prognosis after treatment. Finding testicular cancer at an early point in time is also likely to salvage a man's fertility. In fact, the American Cancer Society recommends that any man who comes across a lump around the testicles should consult a healthcare professional immediately. It's important because testicular cancer is one of the few cancers that can be detected early and nipped in the bud right away.

Who should watch out for testicular cancer?

- Men in the age group of 20-39 years
- Men with a family history of the disease
- Men with an undescended testis (See "The Descent of the Testes," page 21)
- Men who have had a malignant or cancerous testicular tumor in the past

A testicular exam you can do by yourself to check for testicular cancer/lumps

By now, you have probably understood the importance of a testicular self-exam, as well as the requirement for a prompt diagnosis of testicular lumps. So, how do you go about checking your testicles for these infamous lumps? Testicular self-exams have a precise technique, and they are likely to show results only if you follow the respective instructions. In brief, mastering the testicular self-exam to catch a lump as early as possible is the answer to all your worries.

Testicular self-exam

The best time for a testicular self-exam is after you have had a warm bath or shower. This is when the skin of your scrotum is the most relaxed. You want it to be relaxed so you can examine your testicles thoroughly. Here's what you do next:

1. Hold your penis such that it's out of the way.
2. Check one testis at a time.
3. Hold the testicle you are examining between your thumb and fingers with both your hands.
4. Gently roll the testicle you are examining between your fingers.
5. Feel for any hard lumps or bumps around your testicle. Also, look for any variation in size, swelling, or abnormality around the testicle.
6. Repeat the same process for the adjoining testicle.

You can also watch the following videos to help yourself master the technique of testicular self-exams perfectly:

https://youtu.be/T52hM4utM58

https://youtu.be/R1zMar5SRBM

Most of the things you may come across are probably normal. For instance, it's normal if one of your testes is slightly larger than the other one, or if one testicle hangs lower than its neighbor. You are also likely to feel the epididymis (see page 16) as a small swelling on the upper side of each testicle. Additionally, you may feel blood vessels, tubes carrying sperm, and supporting tissue around the testes. You may confuse them for abnormal swellings at first, but these are most likely normal. Repeated testicular self-exams will help you understand what's normal and what's abnormal for your testicles. When in doubt, speak to your doctor.

Celebrities who survived testicular cancer

Here's the good news! Nearly everyone can conquer testicular cancer, just like several of its victims in the past and present. Well, it's a curable disease after all. The prognosis of cancer of the testicles is very good with early detection and prompt treatment. Let's have a look at some of the success stories.

Lance Edward Armstrong

Lance Armstrong is a former professional road-racing cyclist. He won the tour de France medal for seven consecutive years between 1999 and 2005. Armstrong was diagnosed with testicular cancer in 1996 at the young age of 25. He had stage III testicular cancer with metastasis in his lungs, abdomen, and brain. That's how aggressive the disease was by the time it was detected! Symptomatically, he presented with swollen testicles and blood-stained sputum when coughing.

Subsequently, Armstrong underwent his first surgery, a so-called orchiectomy (see page 83), on October 3 to remove his cancer-ridden testicle. This surgery was followed by another one to remove metastasized tumors from his brain on October 25. Additionally, he underwent extensive chemotherapy post-surgery to counter the testicular tumor metastasis and relapse. His last chemo session was on December 13, 1996. After thorough tests, he was declared cancer-free in February, 1997.

Testicular cancer definitely did not put a stop to Armstrong's career. He engaged in training again only to win some more medals and accolades after he conquered this condition in 1997.

Despite his severe disease and subsequent treatment, Lance Armstrong went on to have three children with his first wife, Kristen Richards, with sperm he had banked before he underwent chemotherapy and surgery. In 2008, Armstrong began dating Anna Hansen, with whom he conceived a child naturally, despite speculations about affected fertility due to chemotherapy.

Lance Armstrong did not just rule the tour de France and the cycling world, but he killed stage III testicular cancer to only emerge a winner in all aspects. He also founded the Lance Armstrong Foundation which was later rechristened the 'LiveStrong Foundation.' This institution focuses on promoting cancer research and helping cancer patients deal with this dangerous disease.

As a sad side note, after long investigations against him, Lance Armstrong admitted in January, 2013 to have taken doping substances throughout much of his career. Already a year earlier, he was deprived of all of his titles from 1998 to present.

Tom Green

Tom Green is a Canadian writer, actor, rapper, comedian, media personality, and talk show moderator. He is well known as the host of MTV's Tom Green Show. Tom was diagnosed with testicular cancer in 2000. He underwent several successful surgeries to remove his right testicle and lymph nodes on his right side. This surgery and subsequent chemotherapy sessions managed to cure Tom Green's testicular cancer with an excellent prognosis. In fact, he even resumed his acting career after overcoming his illness.

To increase awareness of testicular cancer among young men, Green recorded a 1-hour special show during his treatment for MTV. It was called The Tom Green Cancer Special and contained footage of his cancer surgery too.

Tom later went on to start the Tom Green's Nuts Cancer Fund to raise funds for cancer research and spread awareness on testicular cancer. He also sang an original song he'd written to encourage young men to perform testicular self-exams.

Steve Scott

Steve Scott was a world-class runner diagnosed with testicular cancer at 38. His cancer was detected when he came across a hardened lump in his testicle. Scott was told that he had a very serious form of testicular cancer. He underwent multiple surgeries and overcame the malignant tumor successfully. To share his experiences with others, Steve Scott wrote his autobiography with the title 'The Miller,' in which he talks about his fight with testicular cancer and the importance of regular testicular self-exams and living healthy.

Tyler Austin

Christopher Tyler Austin is an outfielder for the New York Yankees. He was born on September 6, 1991. The Baseball America ranked Austin the 77th best prospect in baseball, before the 2013 baseball season.

Austin was diagnosed with testicular cancer at a young age of 17. He underwent surgery and extensive treatment for the same and has been cancer-free since then.

Testicular cancer awareness campaigns that have made it to the news

Testicular cancer is curable with a significantly high survival rate when detected early. Hence, celebrities are pitching in with awareness campaigns that are going viral, in addition to the charities that spread awareness about this no-longer-so-deadly disease. Here's a list of some of the most important testicular campaigns and charities that have made it to the news.

LiveStrong Foundation

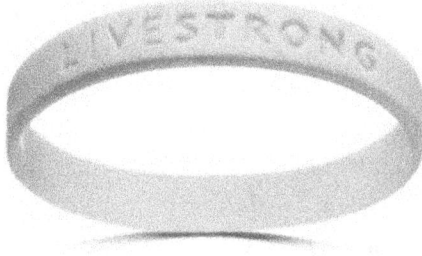

This foundation is synonymous with the yellow LiveStrong wristbands today. Lance Armstrong, himself a testicular cancer survivor, started this foundation. He has brought cancer research and awareness to the forefront with several fundraisers and campaigns focusing on 'Live Strong' to help cancer patients deal with this disease. His efforts have managed to raise more than $250 million for cancer research and support. In fact, the yellow LiveStrong bands alone brought in revenue of more than $55 million.

CARES Initiative (Cancer Alliance for Research, Education, and Survivorship):

Scott Hamilton, a figure skater and Olympic Gold Medalist founded the CARES initiative along with the Cleveland Clinic Taussig Cancer Centre. This is also the same hospital where he himself underwent treatment for testicular cancer. CARES focuses on advancing cancer research and improving the quality of care for cancer patients. Additionally, this organization also acts as a cancer support group by connecting newly diagnosed cancer patients with cancer survivors. Until now, the CARES initiative has managed to raise more than $10 million in funds for cancer research and education.

Check One Two movement's #FeelingNuts campaign

The #FeelingNuts has gone viral on the internet with celebrities grabbing their crotches for a good cause. It is much like the celebrated ice bucket challenge of the ALS foundation, as it aims at creating awareness about regular testicular self-examinations. The campaign tries to encourage young men to examine their "nuts" on a regular basis to be able to detect testicular cancer as soon as possible. So far, Spencer Matthews, Ricky Gervais, Alan Carr, Jack Whitehall, Hugh Jackman, and William Shatner have joined this movement on social media. All one has to do is post the #FeelingNuts with a funny video or picture on a social platform of your choice, and then encourage two more people to take the crotch-grab challenge.

10 Scrotal Conditions likely to Affect the Testes

The scrotum is made up of loose folds of skin at the base of the penis. These scrotal folds form pouches or bags that hold both the testicles inside them. The scrotum is divided into two compartments by a thin partition that keeps both of the testes separated from each other. Thanks to this structural division, pathologies which affect one testicle may not always affect the other one.

The three major ailments of the scrotum are inguinal or scrotal hernia, haematocele, and hydrocele. These conditions may affect either one or both of the scrotal pouches at the same time. Very often, inguinal hernias are accompanied by hydrocele, so it's important to understand both of these medical conditions separately and in combination.

Scrotal/ Inguinal hernia

A scrotal hernia is a hernia (protrusion) in the scrotal region or groin. Your doctor will more correctly refer to this condition as an inguinal hernia or rupture. This condition is actually a passage of tissue or intestines from the abdomen into the scrotal pouches through muscular defects or weakened spots in the pelvic floor. Consequently, a bulge or swelling in the scrotum or groin or on either sides of the pelvic bone is usually the first sign of an inguinal hernia.

Inguinal hernias are 10 times more common in men as compared to women. In fact, the risk of an inguinal hernia is as much as 27% in men and a mere 3% in females [39].

The testes descend down to the scrotum during fetal development through the inguinal canal (see chapter 2, page 7). Normally, the internal inguinal ring is supposed to close once the testes have descended into the scrotum. Sometimes the inguinal canal remains open on one or both sides, increasing one's risk of developing inguinal or scrotal hernias. Under such circumstances, the inguinal canals act like viable openings capable of allowing abdominal contents like muscles and intestines to protrude down to the scrotum in the presence of underlying muscular weaknesses.

Inguinal hernias are classified into 4 groups clinically:

1. _Reversible inguinal hernias:_ In such hernias, the protruding contents can be pushed back into the abdomen with careful and gentle pressure. Such a manual adjustment is only temporary, and the herniating contents may protrude back into the scrotum after a while, if no countermeasures are taken.

2. _Irreducible/ incarcerated hernias:_ These hernias cannot be pushed back into the abdomen with manual pressure alone. They are likely to require surgery for the same.

3. _Obstructed hernia:_ The lumen of the herniated intestinal segment is obstructed in this kind of inguinal hernias. As a result, they tend to be painful and dangerous.

4. _Strangulated hernia:_ The blood supply to the herniated contents gets cut-off resulting in ischemia in strangulated hernias. Such an occurrence is dangerous to say the least, considering the possibility of tissue death around the strangulated intestinal areas.

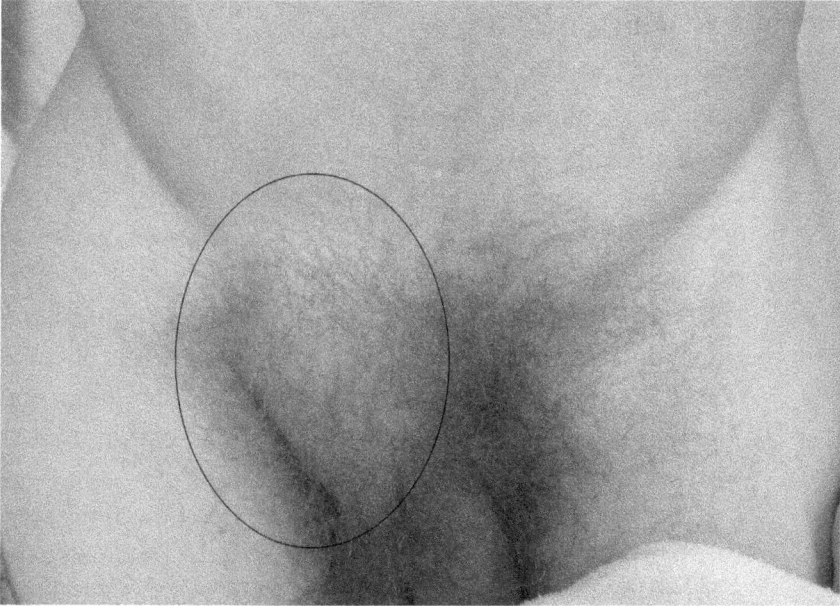

Figure 19: Inguinal hernia
(Source: James Heilman, MD, CC BY-SA 3.0)

The picture shows an inguinal or scrotal hernia on the right side, illustrating how a consequent swelling would appear on the outside.

Causes of inguinal hernia

Generally, heavy lifting, chronic constipation, chronic cough, obesity, and jobs that require manual labor or lifting, and standing for long hours are inclined to increase one's risk of developing inguinal hernias. Chronic constipation tends to weaken the pelvic floor muscles due to repeated straining on the toilet-seat to pass motion. Such factors weaken the pelvic floor and abdominal muscles; hence, increasing the chances of weak spots on the abdominal wall that leave room for herniation of the abdominal contents.

Symptoms of inguinal hernia:

- The primary symptom of inguinal or scrotal hernias is a bulge or swelling in the groin on the affected side. This bulge generally develops over a period of weeks or months.
- The swelling or bulge frequently increases or becomes prominent when coughing, straining for motions, or when standing up.
- The herniating contents often go back into the abdomen when pushed back manually with gentle pressure. Note that the contents are unlikely to move back into the abdomen in irreversible, obstructed, and strangulated hernias.
- A sensation of heaviness, tugging, or burning is common in the region of the bulge. The heaviness and bulge have a propensity to disappear on lying down and increase on bending or standing.
- Inguinal hernias are usually painless. They may become painful if the hernia is of the incarcerated or strangulated type.
- An obstructed or strangulated inguinal hernia may also cause nausea and vomiting.

Diagnosis of inguinal hernias:

A physical examination and thorough history of the complaints is usually sufficient to help diagnose an inguinal hernia. Just examining the bulge or swelling in the groin during coughing, standing, and lying down is often enough to help the healthcare professional confirm an inguinal hernia diagnosis. An ultrasound or further tests are seldom required for the same.

Treatment:

Surgery is the only treatment for inguinal hernias. Hernia repair is also one of the most common surgeries among men. In the United States alone, about 750,000 hernia repair surgeries are carried out each year [40, 41].

Incarcerated and strangulated hernias are likely to result in sudden pain, nausea and vomiting, and more severe complications such as ischemia, gangrene, or obstruction of the herniated segments. Such a situation is a medical emergency calling for immediate surgery. Based on clinical experience, most surgeons recommend elective surgery once an inguinal hernia is detected to avoid obstruction or strangulation and their associated complications.

All the same, most inguinal hernias rarely require surgery. A small painless bulge may remain harmless and asymptomatic for a long time. There is still a possibility of complications, but this isn't a certainty. Fortunately, most of the inguinal hernias do not get obstructed or strangulated. Speak to your doctor to clarify if you require surgery, and if still in doubt, get a second opinion from a different expert.

If the healthcare professionals recommend surgery, then a hernia repair operation (also called herniorraphy) is performed to push the herniated organs back into the abdomen. The weak muscular spots on the pelvic floor are strengthened with a mesh to prevent the reappearance of an inguinal hernia in the future.

Prognosis:

Early treatment with surgery and preventive measures is apt to cure an inguinal hernia. But, there is still some possibility of infection, post-herniorraphy pain syndrome, and scars after hernia repair surgery. To improve the prognosis of an inguinal hernia, with or without surgery, one should follow these simple recommendations:

- Avoid heavy lifting
- Avoid rapid weight gain or weight loss
- Eat a high-fiber diet and drink plenty of water to avoid constipation
- Avoid smoking
- Get a cough treated promptly

- Use scrotal supports or athletic scrotal straps and avoid standing for too long
- Engage in physiotherapy under the guidance of a qualified therapist to gently stimulate and train the respective muscles of your abdomen and pelvis.

Hydrocele

Hydrocele is a collection of fluid in the sac around the testes. Normally, the body produces fluid around the testes that gets absorbed by the adjoining tissues. Yet, certain conditions can result in an excess of fluid production and accumulation in this area, resulting in a hydrocele. This is commonly seen in infants and is bound to disappear by itself within the first year of life. Around 1-2% of boys are born with a hydrocele. Similarly, this condition may also affect boys and men alike regardless of their age. In the older age group, inflammation and injury are the most likely causes of hydroceles.

Most hydroceles themselves are painless, but they are likely to cause scrotal discomfort from an unusually swollen groin. The pain is also expected to aggravate as the swelling and inflammation increases. Sometimes, the swelling is a little less in the mornings and increases in the evenings.

Hydrocele is diagnosed with a physical examination to rule out the other causes of scrotal swelling. A trans-illumination test is performed by shining a torch over the swollen scrotum to check for clear fluid. In addition, an ultrasound of the groin or scrotum may be performed to look for scrotal hernias and other causes of scrotal swellings. Blood tests and urine analysis are recommended to rule out epididymitis and other infections.

Hydrocele is treated with a surgical procedure known as the hydrocelectomy. It aims to drain out the excess fluid collected in the scrotum, easing the discomfort and pain around the groin. Surgery also reduces the complications of hydrocele.

A hydrocele by itself is not dangerous and may hardly cause any severe complications. However, in cases where the hydrocele actually results from an underlying of adjunct causes like testicular tumors, infections, or inguinal hernias, there is a threat of infertility and other complications.

Haematocele

A haematocele is the collection of blood within the scrotal pouches, to differentiate from fluid collected in the case of a hydrocele. Usually, it is more painful than a hydrocele. The most common cause of this swelling is trauma to the groin. The investigations and diagnostic procedures are similar to that of hydrocele (see page 104). Haematoceles are managed with immediate surgery and treatment of the underlying cause or source of bleeding.

11 Prevention is better than Cure: Precluding Testicular Illnesses

The proverbial statement, 'Prevention is better than cure' holds true in most cases. Especially when you look at this idiom in the context of diseases, it speaks mountains of truth. In fact, the very first thought that comes to anyone's mind when one hears about a deadly or annoyingly incurable disease is, 'How do I prevent myself or my family from catching it?'

Prevention does not mean that one can avoid all of the testicular illnesses described in this book, but you can lower the chances and/or severity of their occurrence.

Prevention of testicular infections

Testicular infections like epididymitis (see page 44) and orchitis (see page 49) can be prevented by following a few simple precautionary measures:

- Maintain genital hygiene: Clean the tip of your penis and foreskin thoroughly by pulling the foreskin backwards daily. Also, keep your genitals clean after every visit to the washroom. This will prevent the retrograde or backward entry of microorganisms from your urine and stool into your testes through the urethra.
- Use a condom, especially during sexual intercourse with multiple partners or during anal sex. Since, most testicular infections are from bacteria residing in the anus and genitals, condoms, or other barrier contraceptives are essential to prevent their entry into the urethra. See the section on causes of testicular infections in chapter 6, which starts on page 45 to know more about these bacteria.

Prevention of testicular torsion

Testicular torsion is a spontaneous phenomenon, wherein the testes rotate along with the spermatic cords (see chapter 7, page 52). The presence of an anatomical deformity known as the bell-clapper deformity is its primary cause. The bell-clapper deformity cannot be corrected surgically, nor can it be easily diagnosed. Therefore, you can't prevent this condition from occurring, but if it's treated promptly, the affected testis can be salvaged. A further cause of testicular torsion is trauma, which can happen in the course of accidents or sports. As a preventive measure, sports enthusiasts or athletes should protect their testicles with scrotal supports or jockstraps.

Prevention of testicular trauma and pain

Most sportsmen indulging in aggressive or contact sports like soccer, baseball, cricket, hockey, or martial arts have an increased risk of testicular injury or trauma. Similarly, cyclists and athletes also face a higher chance of such damage. Hence, it's recommended that you use athletic scrotal pads or so-called "cups" to protect your groin from harm. The pads are also useful in preventing testicular pain and swelling, as they provide support to the scrotum and testicles.

Prevention of testicular lumps

For most testicular lumps like varicocele and benign testicular tumors, preventive measures are very limited. At least, avoiding standing for too long or using athletic scrotal pads if your job entails long hours of standing or walking may reduce your risk of varicocele development. Varicoceles are a bunch of loosened veins in the testes (see also page 60). This usually happens due to loss of elasticity of the vessel walls if they have to work against gravity for too long due to too many hours of being on your feet. The scrotal pad provides support to the scrotum and testicles to relieve the pressure of gravity on the veins, thus lowering the likelihood of a varicocele.

Preventing a testicular cyst/ spermatocele can even be a pleasant experience. These lumps are nothing but cystic collections of sperm in the testes. Some experts suggest that having sexual intercourse and/or masturbating regularly may help prevent a spermatocele. For obvious reasons, frequent ejaculations are likely to drain the sperm out of the testes and thus may prevent excess collections of sperm in the testes.

Prevention of scrotal conditions (Inguinal hernias and hydrocele)

Generally, scrotal/ inguinal hernia, haematocele and hydrocele are direct consequences of weak abdominal muscles. Chronic cough, constipation, weight lifting, or heavy lifting is likely to exert increased pressure on the abdominal muscles, and thus, to precipitate inguinal hernias, haematocele and hydrocele. So, getting chronic cough and constipation treated promptly is one way to prevent these conditions by reducing the pressure on your abdominal and pelvic floor muscles. Avoid straining to pass motion and reduce coughing quickly by getting it treated with appropriate medications and other measures such as inhalation of steam, e.g. mixed with an expectorant inhalant.

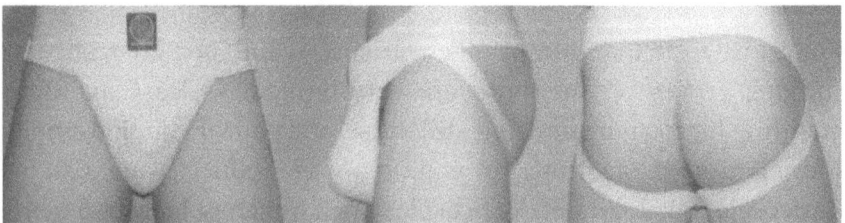

Figure 20: Athletic supporter/ Jockstrap

Weight-lifters and men who have to be on their feet for long hours, including sportsmen, athletes, and dancers should use athletic scrotal pads for support. These pads provide support to the scrotum, consequently reducing the pressure on your abdominal muscles and scrotal muscles. An athletic supporter is also referred to as a jockstrap or posing pouch. The picture above (Figure 20) shows a man wearing an athletic supporter.

Prevention of testicular cancer

Unfortunately, there is no surefire way of preventing testicular cancer, as we still only have limited knowledge about the causes of these dangerous tumors in the testicles. However, healthcare professionals recommend a regular self-examination of one's testes to locate these tumors at the earliest time when they are the most curable. Consult the section, 'A testicular exam you can do by yourself to check for testicular cancer/lumps' on page 93 to learn more about it.

There's more you can do too! Like adjusting your lifestyle and getting the underlying conditions of the testicles treated promptly to reduce your risk of testicular cancer.

General Preventive Measures

1) Examine your testes regularly for lumps and swelling, preferably once a month.

2) Be especially vigilant for testicular lumps if you have a family history or personal history of testicular cancer.

3) If your son or a young boy in the family has cryptorchidism or undescended testes, speak to his doctor about surgical correction to reduce the risk of testicular cancer. Refer to page 21 to learn more about undescended testes.

4) Get any testicular infections like epididymitis and orchitis, or testicular lumps like testicular cysts/ spermatocele, varicocele, and benign testicular tumors treated promptly. Infections and lumps are common predisposing factors for cancers.

5) Limit your intake of alcohol and tobacco to reduce your risk of cancer. If possible, consider quitting smoking entirely, since there is overwhelming scientific evidence that smoking contributes to or directly causes the formation of cancer in various organs. The regular consumption of alcohol is also considered carcinogenic, meaning that it may trigger different types of cancers.

6) Use a condom when indulging in sexual intercourse with multiple partners. Condoms don't prevent testicular cancer, but they prevent dangerous STDs (sexually transmitted diseases) which may cause testicular cancer. Among these are ailments like gonorrhea and syphilis which can result in severe testicular infections or inflammation. Testicular infections are one of the risk factors of testicular cancer.

7) Do not carry a switched-on mobile phone or other radiation-emitting device such as a pager in the pockets of your pants or anywhere near your testes. There is significant scientific evidence that the radio waves of such devices reduce the amount and viability of a man's sperm and increases the risk of developing testicular cancer (see page 78). If you have to use a mobile phone due to your profession or other reasons, then keep it away from your "crown jewels" and consider using a cover that contains a shielding towards the body. You can find commercial products for this purpose by searching for "mobile phone EMF shielding" with an internet search engine. It is also worth considering wearing shielded underpants which you can find, searching for "shielded underwear." Even though it is an ongoing debate and there are different judgements from different experts on the degree of harm caused by radiofrequency electromagnetic radiation (RF-EMF), from

my point of view, the existing scientific literature, which has found harmful effects, suffices to justify the recommendation of taking protective measures. Compared to the concerns, sufferings, and also costs of, for example, infertility or testicular cancer, the comparatively minimal investment into shielding devices and clothing is well justified.

Dietary Preventive measures

Some fruits and vegetables contain anti-oxidants and other beneficial substances which are capable of reducing the cancerous activity within your body. These substances also improve the immune system to help your body improve its disease-fighting capacity. Here's a list of food items you can opt to have regularly to reduce your risk of testicular cancer, or any other cancer for that matter:

Basil is an antioxidant which may prevent cancer. It contains monoterpenes which are beneficial antioxidants, and gives basil its cancer-fighting ability. The holy basil or tulsi, a variant of the basil used for culinary purposes is known for its potent healing properties in Ayurveda. This centuries'-old system of medicine uses this herb in the treatment of different conditions including cancer.

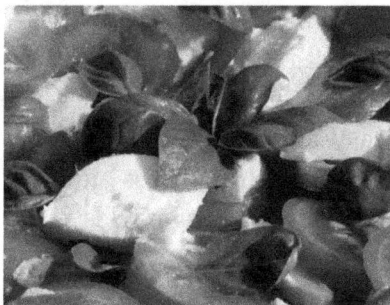

Rosemary, another gastronomic herb contains cancer-preventing properties. Scientific studies show that rosemary is likely to prevent cancer and suppresses tumor growth by up to 46% percent as compared to those who did not ingest it [42]. And it's easy on your palate too; all you have to do is add a few rosemary leaves to your food.

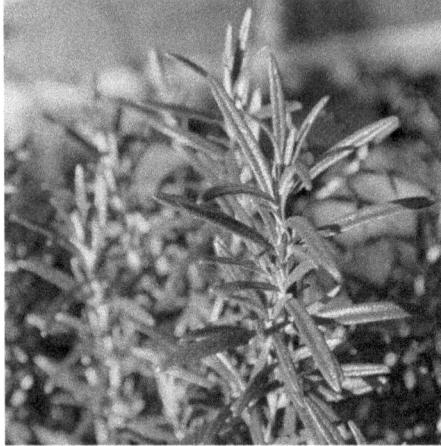

Fresh berries and **Green teas** contain several bioflavonoids which have cancer-inhibiting properties [43]. Green tea also contains essential polyphenols. All of these substances are anti-oxidants and beneficial to your health. Fresh and uncooked onions and apples also contain flavonoids, and thus are recommended as well.

It has been known for a long time that raw **cruciferous vegetables** such as broccoli, brussel sprouts, red cabbage, garden cress, and watercress contain protective substances such as sulphoraphane and isothiocyanates, which help our bodies raise the level of glutathione-S-transferases (GST), which play an important role in the protection against different types of cancer, including testicular ones [44, 45]. An easy and comfortable way of consuming these beneficial substances are raw-press juices, preferably from organically grown, cruciferous vegetables, since these on average contain much less pesticides, etc. You can buy such juices in many health food stores or over the internet.

The researchers Dr. Paul Talalay, Dr. Gary H. Posner, and their colleagues at the Johns Hopkins University, Baltimore have already found, during the 1990s, that sulphoraphane blocks tumor growth [46].

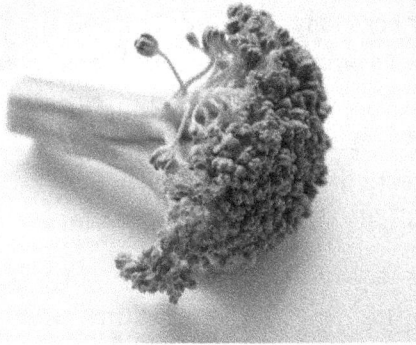

Broccoli is rich in this nutrient, and hence contributes to inhibit the growth of tumors, both benign as well as malignant [47]. Eating it raw or lightly cooked preserves the cancer-inhibiting substances in broccoli. For example, add raw broccoli florets to your salad to benefit from its many health benefits.

One study showed that experimental animals fed on **watercress** were less likely to develop lung cancer despite being exposed to tobacco smoke [48]. **Mustard** and **watercress** are rich in isothiocyanates which are also considered to have cancer-preventing effects.

An Italian study found that individuals who consumed more than 7 servings of **tomatoes** a week had a 60% lower chance of developing colon, stomach, or rectal cancer (because these types of cancers were included in the study) [49]. There is a justified reason to infer that this effect also applies to other forms of cancer including the one that affects the testicles. Tomatoes contain lycopene, which is known to help your body kill mutant cells before they can grow and finally form cancerous tumors.

Sweet red peppers also contain lycopene, so they are good cancer fighters too. On the other hand, hot peppers are high in capsaicin, a phytochemical that is well known for its neutralizing effects on carcinogenic (cancer-causing substances) chemicals like nitrosamines. Capsaicin is also known to block the pain pathways and ease pain when applied locally.

The word "cancer" is most likely to press the panic button in most of our minds. However, being vigilant towards one's body and testicular health could go a long way in helping to prevent testicular cancer. Although it is important to take a few preventive measures for testicular cancer, the key to overcoming this disease is EARLY DETECTION. That is the best you can do for your testicles.

Not just in the case of testicular cancer, but early detection of most testicular conditions can prevent unwanted complications and long-term consequences like infertility, chronic testicular infections, or even removal of one or both testes due to testicular cancer.

All said and done, I hope that you can use the information provided in this book to stay calm and at the same time be attentive to your testicles. It is an important measure of precaution to select and consult a physician specialized in the field of urology, and to build a trusting relationship with him/her. This way, you already know with whom to turn to in case you need to be treated promptly for whatever testicular condition you may experience.

12 Specialized Urology Treatment Centers Around the World

Urologists treat testicular illnesses. Urology is a branch of medicine that deals with the male and female urinary system and the male reproductive organs. It is also referred to as genitourinary surgery. The organs covered by Urology are the male and female kidneys, adrenal glands, ureters, urinary bladder, urethra, testes, epididymis, Vas Deferens, seminal vesicles, bulbourethral or Cowper's glands, prostate gland, and the penis. Testicular cancer is treated by a urologist or urosurgeon and an oncologist.

The following is a list of renowned medical facilities around the world with excellent urology services, though this list may not be complete (as of April 2018):

North America

- Cleveland Clinic, Cleveland, OH
- Mayo Clinic, Rochester, MN
- Johns Hopkins Hospital, Baltimore, MD
- UCLA Medical Centre, Los Angeles, CA
- New York-Presbyterian University Hospital of Columbia and Cornell, New York, NY
- UCSF Medical Center, San Francisco, CA
- Duke University Hospital, Durham, NC
- Hospitals of the University of Pennsylvania-Penn Presbyterian, Philadelphia, PA
- Memorial Sloan Kettering Cancer Centre, New York, NY and Northwestern Memorial Hospital, Chicago, IL
- False Creek Healthcare Centre, Vancouver, Canada
- Rockyview Urology Clinic, Calgary, Canada
- Clinique Medic Elle, Quebec, Canada

Latin America

- Hospital Sao Rafael, Sao Paulo, Brazil
- Hospital Samaritano de Sao Paulo, Sao Paulo, Brazil
- Hospital Velmar, Ensenada, Mexico
- Hospital CIMA Monterrey, Monterrey, Mexico
- San Angel Hospital, Nuevo Laredo, Mexico
- Hospital El Cruce, Buenos Aires, Argentina
- Hospital Italiano des Buenos Aires, Argentina
- Hospital Clínico de la Universidad de Chile, Santiago de Chile
- Clínica Alemana de Santiago de Chile, Santiago de Chile
- Hospital Universitario San José de Popyan, Popayan, Columbia

Europe and Middle East

UK

- Scarborough General Hospital, Scarborough, North Yorkshire
- Herts and Essex Urology Clinic, Capio Rivers Hospital, Sawbridgeworth
- Hertford Clinic, Hertfordshire
- Holly House Hospital, Buckhursthill, Essex
- BUPA Roding Hospital, Ilford, Essex
- London Urology Associates, Princess Grace Hospital, 47 Nottingham Place, London
- London Urology Centre, 69 Wimpole Street, London
- North London Nuffield Hospital, Enfield, Middlesex
- London Independent Hospital, 1 Beaumont Square, London
- BUPA Hartswood Hospital, Brentwood, Essex

Germany

- University Medical Center Hamburg-Eppendorf, University Hospital, Hamburg
- Klinikum Stuttgart, Public Hospital, Stuttgart
- Heidelberg University Hospital, Heidelberg
- Humboldt Klinikum, Berlin
- St. Hedwig Hospital, Berlin
- University Hospital Münster, Urology Clinic, Münster
- Technical University Munich, Klinikum rechts der Isar, Urology Clinic, Munich
- Ludwig-Maximilian-University Munich, Klinikum Großhadern, Urology Clinic, Munich
- University Hospital, Urology Clinic, Freiburg
- St.-Antonius-Hospital, Urology Clinic, Eschweiler

France

- Clinique Saint-Augustin, Bordeaux
- GH Lariboisiere-Fernand Widal, Paris
- Hopital La Timone Adultes, Marseille
- Hopital Prive Saint-Martin, Pessac
- Institut Mutualiste Montsouris, Paris
- Hopital Prive Clairval, Marseille
- Clinique Saint Jean Languedoc, Toulouse
- CLCC Oscar-Lambret, Lille

Spain

- IDCSalud Hospital General de Catalunya
- Hospital Internacional Medimar
- Sanitas Hospitales, Madrid
- HM Hospitales, Madrid
- Sant Joan de Déu-Barcelona Children's Hospital, Barcelona
- Clinica La Luz, Madrid
- Vithas Xanit International Hospital, Malaga
- Nisa Pardo de Aravaca Hospital, Madrid
- Corposalud Clinic, Valencia

- Quirón Madrid University Hospital, Madrid

Portugal

- British Hospital Lisbon XXI, Lisbon

Greece

- Hygeia Hospital, Athens
- MITERA General, Maternity-Gynecology & Children's Hospital, Athens

Turkey

- Acibadem Maslak Hospital,
- Medipol Mega Hospital, Istanbul
- Anadolu Medical Center, Gabze
- Liv Hospital, Istanbul
- International Hospital, Istanbul

Israel

- Hadassah University Medical Center, Israel
- Herzliya Medical Center, Israel
- Assuta Hospital, Israel
- Rabin Medical Center, Israel

Asia-Pacific

Australia

- Brisbane Urology Clinic, Brisbane
- Royal Melbourne Hospital, Melbourne
- Calvary John James Hospital, Canberra
- Japinder Khosa Paediatric Surgery, Perth
- Mackay Base Hospital, Mackay
- Sydney Prostate Cancer Centre, Sydney

Asia

- Bangkok Hospital, Pattaya, Thailand
- Bumrungrad Hospital, Bangkok, Thailand

- BNH Hospital, Bangkok, Thailand
- Raffles Hospital, Singapore
- Tan Tock Seng Hospital, Singapore
- Gleneagles Hospital, Singapore
- Mount Elizabeth Hospital, Singapore
- Columbia Asia Hospitals, Bangalore, India
- Apollo Hospital, Chennai, India
- Moolchand Medcity, New Delhi, India
- Fortis Hospitals, India
- Sevenhills Hospital, Mumbai, India
- KPJ Tawakkal Specialist Hospital, Malaysia
- Mahkota Medical Centre, Malaysia
- KPJ Ampang Puteri Specialist Hospital, Malaysia
- Gleneagles Intan Medical Centre, Malaysia
- KPJ Damansara Specialist Hospital, Malaysia
- Sunway Medical Centre, Malaysia

South Africa

- Da Vinci Cancer Robotic Surgery Centre, Cape Town, South Africa
- Dr. Paul Whitaker, Cape Town, South Africa
- Arwyp Medical Centre, Gauteng, South Africa
- Lenmed Clinic, Johannesburg, South Africa
- Zuid Afrikaans Hospital, pretoria, South Africa
- Wilmed Park Private Hospital, North West Province , Klerksdorp, South Africa
- Hibiscus Private Hospital, KwaZulu Natal, South Africa
- Geneva Clinic, Western Cape, South Africa
- Bay View Private Hospital, Mossel Bay, South Africa
- Groote Schuur Hospital, Western Cape, South Africa

13 References and Links

1. Testicular cancer incidence statistics : Cancer Research UK. (n.d.). Retrieved April 18, 2015, from http://www.cancerresearchuk.org/cancer-info/cancerstats/types/testis/incidence/uk-testicular-cancer-incidence-statistics

2. Gilbert, S. F. (2000). *Developmental biology* (6th ed.). Sunderland, Mass: Sinauer Associates.

3. Sadler, T. W., & Langman, J. (2012). *Langman's medical embryology* (12th ed.). Philadelphia: Wolters Kluwer Health/Lippincott Williams & Wilkins.

4. Berkowitz, G. S., Lapinski, R. H., Dolgin, S. E., Gazella, J. G., Bodian, C. A., & Holzman, I. R. (1993). Prevalence and natural history of cryptorchidism. *Pediatrics*, 92(1), 44–49.

5. Eddy, E. (2006). The spermatozoon. *Knobil and Neill's physiology of reproduction, 1*, 3–54.

6. Barada, J. H., Weingarten, J. L., & Cromie, W. J. (1989). Testicular salvage and age-related delay in the presentation of testicular torsion. *The Journal of Urology, 142*(3), 746–748.

7. Ringdahl, E., & Teague, L. (2006). Testicular torsion. *American Family Physician, 74*(10), 1739–1743.

8. Jh, B., Jl, W., & Wj, C. (1989). Testicular salvage and age-related delay in the presentation of testicular torsion. *The Journal of urology, 142*(3), 746–748.

9. UK, C. R. (2014, November 11). Testicular cancer symptoms. Document. Retrieved April 14, 2015, from http://www.cancerresearchuk.org/about-

cancer/type/testicular-cancer/about/testicular-cancer-symptoms

10. Zuniga, A., Lawrentschuk, N., & Jewett, M. A. S. (2010). Organ-sparing approaches for testicular masses. *Nature Reviews Urology, 7*(8), 454–464. doi:10.1038/nrurol.2010.100

11. Elmore, S. (2007). Apoptosis: A Review of Programmed Cell Death. *Toxicologic pathology, 35*(4), 495–516. doi:10.1080/01926230701320337

12. Whitworth, P. W., Pak, C. C., Esgro, J., Kleinerman, E. S., & Fidler, I. J. (1990). Macrophages and cancer. *Cancer Metastasis Reviews, 8*(4), 319–351.

13. What are the key statistics about testicular cancer? (n.d.). Retrieved April 15, 2015, from http://www.cancer.org/cancer/testicularcancer/detailedguide/testicular-cancer-key-statistics

14. Manecksha, R. P., & Fitzpatrick, J. M. (2009). Epidemiology of testicular cancer. *BJU International, 104*(9b), 1329–1333. doi:10.1111/j.1464-410X.2009.08854.x

15. Chien, F. L., Schwartz, S. M., & Johnson, R. H. (2014). Increase in testicular germ cell tumor incidence among Hispanic adolescents and young adults in the United States. *Cancer, 120*(17), 2728–2734. doi:10.1002/cncr.28684

16. Shanmugalingam, T., Soultati, A., Chowdhury, S., Rudman, S., & Van Hemelrijck, M. (2013). Global incidence and outcome of testicular cancer. *Clinical Epidemiology, 5*, 417–427. doi:10.2147/CLEP.S34430

17. Information for Undertanding Testicular Cancer. (n.d.). Retrieved April 18, 2015, from http://www.testicularcancersociety.org/understanding_testicular_cancer.html

18. Herrinton, L. J., Zhao, W., & Husson, G. (2003). Management of cryptorchism and risk of testicular cancer. *American Journal of Epidemiology, 157*(7), 602–605.

19. Choices, N. H. S. (2014, April 7). Testicular Cancer - Symptoms - NHS Choices. Retrieved January 8, 2015, from http://www.nhs.uk/Conditions/Cancer-of-the-testicle/Pages/Symptoms.aspx

20. Li, N., Hauser, R., Holford, T., Zhu, Y., Zhang, Y., Bassig, B. A., … Zheng, T. (2015). Muscle-building supplement use and increased risk of testicular germ cell cancer in men from Connecticut and Massachusetts. *British Journal of Cancer, 112*(7), 1247–1250. doi:10.1038/bjc.2015.26

21. Lacson, J. C. A., Carroll, J. D., Tuazon, E., Castelao, E. J., Bernstein, L., & Cortessis, V. K. (2012). Population-based case-control study of recreational drug use and testis cancer risk confirms an association between marijuana use and nonseminoma risk: Marijuana, Cocaine, and Testicular Tumors. *Cancer, 118*(21), 5374–5383. doi:10.1002/cncr.27554

22. Garaj-Vrhovac, V., Fucić, A., & Horvat, D. (1992). The correlation between the frequency of micronuclei and specific chromosome aberrations in human lymphocytes exposed to microwave radiation in vitro. *Mutation Research, 281*(3), 181–186.

23. Vijayalaxmi, null, Bisht, K. S., Pickard, W. F., Meltz, M. L., Roti Roti, J. L., & Moros, E. G. (2001). Chromosome damage and micronucleus formation in human blood lymphocytes exposed in vitro to radiofrequency radiation at a cellular telephone frequency (847.74 MHz, CDMA). *Radiation Research, 156*(4), 430–432.

24. Villeneuve, P. J., Agnew, D. A., Johnson, K. C., Mao, Y., & Canadian Cancer Registries Epidemiology Research Group. (2002). Brain cancer and occupational exposure to magnetic fields among men: results from a Canadian population-

based case-control study. *International Journal of Epidemiology, 31*(1), 210–217.

25. La Vignera, S., Condorelli, R. A., Vicari, E., D'Agata, R., & Calogero, A. E. (2012). Effects of the exposure to mobile phones on male reproduction: a review of the literature. *Journal of Andrology, 33*(3), 350–356. doi:10.2164/jandrol.111.014373

26. Kesari, K. K., Kumar, S., Nirala, J., Siddiqui, M. H., & Behari, J. (2013). Biophysical evaluation of radiofrequency electromagnetic field effects on male reproductive pattern. *Cell Biochemistry and Biophysics, 65*(2), 85–96. doi:10.1007/s12013-012-9414-6

27. Information for Undertanding Testicular Cancer. (n.d.). Retrieved April 15, 2015, from http://www.testicularcancersociety.org/understanding_testicular_cancer.html

28. Testicular cancer: MedlinePlus Medical Encyclopedia. (n.d.). Retrieved April 15, 2015, from http://www.nlm.nih.gov/medlineplus/ency/article/001288.htm

29. Ayurveda herbal testis cancer cure, Cancer treatment through Ayurveda. DARF. (n.d.). Retrieved April 18, 2015, from http://www.ayurveda-cancer.org/cancerbysystem15.htm

30. Ayurveda herbal testis cancer cure, Cancer treatment through Ayurveda. DARF. (n.d.). Retrieved April 15, 2015, from http://www.ayurveda-cancer.org/cancerbysystem15.htm

31. Blomberg Jensen, M., Jørgensen, A., Nielsen, J. E., Steinmeyer, A., Leffers, H., Juul, A., & Rajpert-De Meyts, E. (2012). Vitamin D metabolism and effects on pluripotency genes and cell differentiation in testicular germ cell tumors in vitro and in vivo. *Neoplasia (New York, N.Y.), 14*(10), 952–963.

32. Kim, Y., & Je, Y. (2014). Vitamin D intake, blood 25(OH)D levels, and breast cancer risk or mortality: a meta-analysis. *British Journal of Cancer, 110*(11), 2772–2784. doi:10.1038/bjc.2014.175

33. Maalmi, H., Ordóñez-Mena, J. M., Schöttker, B., & Brenner, H. (2014). Serum 25-hydroxyvitamin D levels and survival in colorectal and breast cancer patients: systematic review and meta-analysis of prospective cohort studies. *European Journal of Cancer (Oxford, England: 1990), 50*(8), 1510–1521. doi:10.1016/j.ejca.2014.02.006

34. Ma, Y., Zhang, P., Wang, F., Yang, J., Liu, Z., & Qin, H. (2011). Association between vitamin D and risk of colorectal cancer: a systematic review of prospective studies. *Journal of Clinical Oncology: Official Journal of the American Society of Clinical Oncology, 29*(28), 3775–3782. doi:10.1200/JCO.2011.35.7566

35. Chen, Q., Espey, M. G., Krishna, M. C., Mitchell, J. B., Corpe, C. P., Buettner, G. R., … Levine, M. (2005). Pharmacologic ascorbic acid concentrations selectively kill cancer cells: action as a pro-drug to deliver hydrogen peroxide to tissues. *Proceedings of the National Academy of Sciences of the United States of America, 102*(38), 13604–13609. doi:10.1073/pnas.0506390102

36. Du, J., Cullen, J. J., & Buettner, G. R. (2012). Ascorbic acid: chemistry, biology and the treatment of cancer. *Biochimica Et Biophysica Acta, 1826*(2), 443–457. doi:10.1016/j.bbcan.2012.06.003

37. Min, Z., Wang, L., Jin, J., Wang, X., Zhu, B., Chen, H., & Cheng, Y. (2014). Pyrroloquinoline Quinone Induces Cancer Cell Apoptosis via Mitochondrial-Dependent Pathway and Down-Regulating Cellular Bcl-2 Protein Expression. *Journal of Cancer, 5*(7), 609–624. doi:10.7150/jca.9002

38. Moen, I., & Stuhr, L. E. B. (2012). Hyperbaric oxygen therapy and cancer—a review. *Targeted Oncology, 7*(4), 233–242. doi:10.1007/s11523-012-0233-x

39. Jenkins, J. T., & O'Dwyer, P. J. (2008). Inguinal hernias. *BMJ, 336*(7638), 269–272. doi:10.1136/bmj.39450.428275.AD

40. Rutkow, I. M., & Robbins, A. W. (1993). Demographic, classificatory, and socioeconomic aspects of hernia repair in the United States. *The Surgical Clinics of North America, 73*(3), 413–426.

41. Classification, clinical features and diagnosis of inguinal and femoral hernias in adults. (n.d.). Retrieved April 18, 2015, from http://www.uptodate.com/contents/classification-clinical-features-and-diagnosis-of-inguinal-and-femoral-hernias-in-adults

42. Petiwala, S. M., Berhe, S., Li, G., Puthenveetil, A. G., Rahman, O., Nonn, L., & Johnson, J. J. (2014). Rosemary (Rosmarinus officinalis) Extract Modulates CHOP/GADD153 to Promote Androgen Receptor Degradation and Decreases Xenograft Tumor Growth. *PLoS ONE, 9*(3). doi:10.1371/journal.pone.0089772

43. Landis-Piwowar, K. R., Milacic, V., & Dou, Q. P. (2008). Relationship between the methylation status of dietary flavonoids and their growth-inhibitory and apoptosis-inducing activities in human cancer cells. *Journal of cellular biochemistry, 105*(2), 514–523. doi:10.1002/jcb.21853

44. Steinkellner, H., Rabot, S., Freywald, C., Nobis, E., Scharf, G., Chabicovsky, M., … Kassie, F. (2001). Effects of cruciferous vegetables and their constituents on drug metabolizing enzymes involved in the bioactivation of DNA-reactive dietary carcinogens. *Mutation Research, 480-481*, 285–297.

45. Tang, L., Zhang, Y., Jobson, H. E., Li, J., Stephenson, K. K., Wade, K. L., & Fahey, J. W. (2006). Potent activation of

mitochondria-mediated apoptosis and arrest in S and M phases of cancer cells by a broccoli sprout extract. *Molecular Cancer Therapeutics, 5*(4), 935–944. doi:10.1158/1535-7163.MCT-05-0476

46. Zhang, Y., Kensler, T. W., Cho, C. G., Posner, G. H., & Talalay, P. (1994). Anticarcinogenic activities of sulforaphane and structurally related synthetic norbornyl isothiocyanates. *Proceedings of the National Academy of Sciences of the United States of America, 91*(8), 3147–3150.

47. Angier, N. (1994, April 12). Benefits of Broccoli Confirmed as Chemical Blocks Tumors. *The New York Times*. Retrieved from http://www.nytimes.com/1994/04/12/science/benefits-of-broccoli-confirmed-as-chemical-blocks-tumors.html

48. Hecht, S. S., Chung, F. L., Richie, J. P., Akerkar, S. A., Borukhova, A., Skowronski, L., & Carmella, S. G. (1995). Effects of watercress consumption on metabolism of a tobacco-specific lung carcinogen in smokers. *Cancer Epidemiology, Biomarkers & Prevention: A Publication of the American Association for Cancer Research, Cosponsored by the American Society of Preventive Oncology, 4*(8), 877–884.

49. Giovannucci, E. (1999). Tomatoes, Tomato-Based Products, Lycopene, and Cancer: Review of the Epidemiologic Literature. *JNCI Journal of the National Cancer Institute, 91*(4), 317–331. doi:10.1093/jnci/91.4.317

14 Glossary

Cancer: A disease caused by uncontrolled and rapid division of abnormal cells in a particular region of the body.

Epididymitis: Infection or inflammation of one or both Epididymis.

Hydrocele: The accumulation of serous fluid in a body sac or cavity.

Haematocele: The accumulation of blood in a body sac or cavity.

Inguinal/ Scrotal Hernia: A medical condition that constitutes the protrusion of the intestinal tissues into the scrotum through the inguinal canal, resulting in a swelling in the groin.

Orchitis: Inflammation or infection of one or both testicles.

Lumps: A compact mass with or without a definite shape and border

Spermatocele: A cyst or fluid-filled swelling in the testis.

Swelling: An abnormal enlargement of a region or part of the body.

Infection: A medical condition that constitutes the entry and multiplication of microorganisms such as bacteria, viruses, and parasites into the body that is normally absent.

Testicular Cancer: Cancer that forms in the tissues of one or both the testes.

Testicular Torsion: A medical condition that involves the twisting of the spermatic cord that holds the testis in the scrotum.

Tumors: A swelling of a region of the body caused by abnormal growth of a tissue, benign or malignant.

Varicocele: A collection or mass of varicose veins in the spermatic cord.

15 Index

16 Photo and image credits

Figure 1: The Male Reproductive System, page 9
Source: by Elf Sternberg, CC BY-SA 3.0,
http://commons.wikimedia.org/wiki/File:Male_anatomy.png

Figure 2: Cross-section of the penis, page 10
Source: by Mcstrother, CC BY 3.0,
http://commons.wikimedia.org/wiki/File:Penis_cross_section.svg

Figure 3: Scrotum and Testis, page 12
Source: Public Domain,
http://commons.wikimedia.org/wiki/File:Illu_testis_1b.jpg

Figure 4: Size of an adult male's testicle, page 13
Source: by Richiex, CC BY-SA 3.0,
http://commons.wikimedia.org/wiki/File:Average_sized_post-
pubertal_testicle.JPG

Figure 5: Inner structure of the testes, page 15
Source: by Cancer Research UK, CC BY-SA 4.0,

Figure 6: Histological section of a testis, page 16
Source: by Doc. RN Dr. Josef Reischig, CSc., CC BY-SA 3.0,
http://commons.wikimedia.org/wiki/File%3ATesticles_(26_2_11)_Cross-
section.jpg

Figure 7: Testis and Epididymis, page 17
Source: Public Domain,
http://commons.wikimedia.org/wiki/File:Illu_testis_surface.jpg#mediavie
wer/File:Illu_testis_surface.jpg

Figure 8: The Prostate gland in relation to its adjacent organs, page 19,
Source: Public Domain,
http://commons.wikimedia.org/wiki/File:Prostatelead.jpg

Figure 9: Scrotum in relaxed and tense state, page 23
Source: By 123GLGL (Own work), CC BY-SA 3.0,
http://commons.wikimedia.org/wiki/File:HQ_SAM_ST2.jpg

Figure 10: Four stages of spermatogenesis, page 25
Source: by Anchor207 (Own work), CC BY-SA 3.0 -

http://commons.wikimedia.org/wiki/File:Spermatogenesis.svg#mediavie
wer/File:Spermatogenesis.svg

Figure 11: Spermatogenesis in the Testis, page 25
Source: by Henry Gray (1918), Public Domain,
http://commons.wikimedia.org/wiki/File:Gray1150.png#mediaviewer/Fil
e:Gray1150.png

Figure 12: Androgenic hair patterns due to testosterone, page 27
Source: I, Genesis89, CC BY-SA 3.0,
http://commons.wikimedia.org/wiki/File:Malepuberty.jpg#mediaviewer/
File:Malepuberty.jpg

Figure, page 31
Source: iStockPhoto

Figure 13: Testicular Torsion, page 52
Source: OpenI,
http://openi.nlm.nih.gov/imgs/512/94/2859224/2859224_431_2009_1096_F
ig1_HTML.png

Figure 14: Schematic picture of a varicocele on the left side (from patient
perspective), page 62
Source: OpenI,
http://openi.nlm.nih.gov/imgs/512/239/3583174/3583174_cln-68-s1-027-
g001.png

Figure 15: Picture of a big varicocele which is clearly visible through the
scrotal skin, page 64
Source: OpenI,
http://openi.nlm.nih.gov/imgs/512/86/3093801/3093801_cln-66-04-691-
g002.png

Figure 16: Adult male with severe gynaecomastia, page 68
Source: By JMZ1122 Dr. Mordcai Blau www.gynecomastia-md.com
(Own work), CC BY-SA 3.0,

Figure 17: Testicular cancer incidence and mortality in 10 countries, page
74
Source: OpenI,
http://openi.nlm.nih.gov/imgs/512/319/3804606/3804606_clep-5-
417Fig1.png

Figure 18: CT scan of a testicular tumor on the left side (see arrow), page 81
Source: OpenI,
http://openi.nlm.nih.gov/imgs/512/50/3977168/3977168_rt-2014-1-5079-g002.png

Picture "Feel your balls," page 92
Source: http://feelyourballstoday.org/site/Facts_pg_4.html

Picture of Livestrong wristband, page 97
Source: By Suuz80 (Own work) [Public domain], via Wikimedia Commons

Figure 19: Inguinal hernia, page 101
Source: By James Heilman, MD (Own work), CC BY-SA 3.0,
http://commons.wikimedia.org/wiki/Category:Inguinal_hernia#mediaviewer/File:Hernia.JPG

Figure 20: Athletic supporter/ Jockstrap, page 108
Source: Public Domain,
http://commons.wikimedia.org/wiki/File:Jockstrap_Front,_Side_and_Rear.jpg#mediaviewer/File:Jockstrap_Front,_Side_and_Rear.jpg

Pictures of different food, pages 111 to 113,
Source: http://www.pixabay.com

www.ingramcontent.com/pod-product-compliance
Lightning Source LLC
Chambersburg PA
CBHW050351280326
41933CB00010BA/1422